Epilepsy after
Non-missile Head Injuries

Epilepsy after Non-missile Head Injuries

BRYAN JENNETT, M.D., F.R.C.S.

Professor of Neurosurgery
The Institute of Neurological Sciences, Glasgow
and The University of Glasgow

Second Edition

WILLIAM HEINEMANN MEDICAL BOOKS LTD
LONDON

First published 1962
entitled Epilepsy after Blunt Head Injuries
Second edition (reset) 1975

ISBN 0 433 17303 3

Printed in Great Britain by
The Whitefriars Press Ltd., London and Tonbridge

CONTENTS

Part I The Problem

Part II The Investigation

Part III Conclusions

FOREWORD

Until 1954, when there was published posthumously Gilbert Phillips' study on traumatic epilepsy occurring after "closed" head injuries in soldiers, there had been no statistical assessment of the frequency with which it occurred, its type, and prognosis. Before this study the subject was befogged by impressions and assertions. Yet it has profound import, not only for diagnosis and treatment, but especially for prognosis in the medico-legal field.

This monograph, which is since Phillips' work the first serious attempt to evaluate the problem of traumatic epilepsy in blunt head injuries, is based on an extensive experience in Oxford, Cardiff and Manchester. Three hundred and eighty one patients, conforming to the definition of "blunt head injuries" followed by epilepsy, have been intensively studied. The influence on the incidence of both early and late epilepsy of a large number of factors are analysed, e.g. of linear and depressed fractures and their sites, of dural penetration, of haematomas, of age, etc., and there is an assessment of the type and the severity of the epilepsy suffered. The series of tables embodying these analyses will be of inestimable value to those who have to deal with the problems arising from head injuries.

Professor Jennett presents essentially a factual report. He attempts little speculative interpretation. His is a study in depth. It is both retrospective and prospective, for many of his patients have been followed for more than four years.

There is a rare and enviable quality and clarity in Professor Jennett's prose, and he has been singularly successful in finding the apt quotation for his chapter headings.

Since I guided the author's first steps in neurology, I may be forgiven a paternal pride in this, the latest, expression of an unusually penetrating and analytical mind, which is satisfied only by the best.

1962   Cohen of Birkenhead

PREFACE TO THE FIRST EDITION

This study began in 1955 at the suggestion of Mr. Walpole Lewin who was then responsible for the care of patients with head injury at the Radcliffe Infirmary, Oxford. His insistence on a high standard of observation and documentation of all head injuries admitted to the Accident Service over the preceding years had made available a series of cases unique in civilian experience. Not only were there 1,000 consecutive injuries but these cases were largely unselected and there was a wealth of clinical information about every one. An analysis of this series and of the patients in it who developed epilepsy brought many interesting facts to light, especially about fits which occur soon after injury (Jennett and Lewin, 1960).

However, the small number who suffered from this complication limited the extent to which the interaction of various factors could be explored, particularly in relation to epilepsy of late onset; and no attempt was made to deal with the material statistically. The need to investigate a larger number of patients with traumatic epilepsy after blunt injuries was obvious, and prompted me to collect additional cases over the succeeding five years, first in Oxford and later in the Cardiff and Manchester Royal Infirmaries. This monograph is based on 381 patients with epilepsy after injury, including the original 64 from Oxford.

I am grateful to Mr. Lewin not only for setting me off on this task but for allowing me to include here the results of our analysis of his series. The Editor of the Journal of Neurology, Neurosurgery and Psychiatry gave permission for the reproduction of Table C3. The Editor of the Annals of the Royal College of Surgeons has kindly allowed me to include material which was the basis of a Hunterian Lecture earlier this year.

I am indebted to several senior colleagues who allowed me to study the records of patients under their care: Mr. J. C. Scott and Mr. Joe Pennybacker in Oxford, Mr. Charles Langmaid and Professor Lambert Rogers in Cardiff and Mr. Richard Johnson and Mr. John Potter in Manchester.

Others have helped more directly with the preparation of this text. Miss Sheila Nicholson of the Radcliffe Infirmary brought resourcefulness and good humour to the problem of following up patients in the Oxford series. Mr. John Darroch of the Statistical Laboratory in the University of Manchester advised me on the preparation of the tables. Mr. Ted Smith of the Department of Medical Illustration in Manchester executed the histogram showing the sources of the series of patients studied. Miss Clare

Bainbridge of the E.E.G. Department, Manchester Royal Infirmary, helped immensely with collecting and classifying information from many records. Dr. Sheila Jennett criticized the typescript as only a wife could; Mr. Robert Tym took on the tiresome task of correcting the proofs as only a good friend would. I am grateful to all of them for the help they have so freely given.

B.J.

PREFACE TO THE SECOND EDITION

It continues to surprise me that the first edition of this book was as well received as it was because, although it provided information not previously available, its presentation now seems to me to have been unnecessarily complicated. Mainly this was because the numbers were so often below the limits for statistical significance that alternative ways of presenting the data were sought in order to confirm suspected correlations. Since it was published many more cases have been collected, with the deliberate intention of expanding the size of the groups with factors which the initial study had shown to be important determinants of late epilepsy. Moving to Glasgow provided me with a new population to explore and it has been reassuring to discover a close correspondence between the findings in the Scottish as compared with the English series. Fortunately the addition of several hundred cases has not altered any of the main conclusions drawn in the first edition, but the findings now stand on a much firmer statistical basis. This has enabled a simpler presentation although more information is available.

Publication of late surveys of World War II combat injuries, and more recently of survivors of the Korean campaign, has prompted the extension of the comparison between missile and non-missile injuries. The concern of paediatricians to know whether young children behave differently in regard to traumatic epilepsy, as they do in most other forms of symptomatic epilepsy, has prompted me to set out separately the data for children under five, as well as to make more extensive comparisons between adults and children (taking 16 years as the watershed). The analysis of EEG data has been simplified because it has become clear to me that there is no consensus among neurologists about what abnormalities in the record should be interpreted as indicating epileptic activity. At the same time, the availability of larger numbers has enabled a study to be made of serial records in order to determine the significance of changes over time. Dr. I. D. Melville kindly assisted with interpretation.

The increasing size of the series has necessitated the use of computers for data processing, and I am grateful to the Computer Servicing Department of the University of Glasgow (Dr. Browning). The way in which the data has been treated and presented owes much to Dr. Robin Knill-Jones of the Department of Medicine in Relation to Computing and Mathematics in Glasgow (Professor W. I. Card), and to Mr. Derek Teather,

M.Sc. of the Department of Statistics and Computer Science at University College London (Professor D. V. Lindley). Financial support has been provided at various stages in the investigation by the British Epilepsy Association, the National Fund for Research into Crippling Diseases and the Royal College of Physicians of London.

The key person in the analysis of this greatly enlarged series has been my Research Assistant, Miss Susan Bennie, B.Sc., whose cheerfulness and persistence has sustained all concerned with this study. My secretaries Mrs. Sally Brown and Mrs. Margaret Smith have coped with what must have been a typist's nightmare — a text with more figures than words.

B.J.

Chapter 1

INTRODUCTION

"It has been asserted almost universally that trauma may cause
epilepsy; I have never been able to understand why."

A. Kinnier Wilson (1923)

The literature teems with widely varying estimates of the frequency with
which epilepsy and head injury are associated, an association which has
been suspected since Hippocratic times (Temkin, 1945). Penetrating
missile injuries are frequently followed by fits and there are many
competent studies of such injuries, most of them dealing with war-injured
men, who form a captive population for follow-up because they remain
traceable through Government agencies for long periods after injury. By
contrast most reports of epilepsy after non-missile head injuries of civilian
life are fragmentary both in regard to observation in the acute stage and to
follow-up. Symonds (1935), in a valuable paper based on only a handful of
cases, posed, but was unable to answer, most of the important questions
about epilepsy after this kind of trauma. He said that an enquiry into the
rate of incidence in patients with closed injuries would be of value but
would have to cover a large number of patients. It is surprising that no one
should have accepted seriously the challenge to provide answers to his
question, so that some years later Garland (1942) could remark that a
good deal of what has been written about traumatic epilepsy was the result
of clinical impression and speculation, but that there was a maximum of
fact and a minimum of speculation concerning epilepsy after gunshot
wounds. Thirty years after that Rapport and Penry (1973) wrote that
criteria for identifying which head-injured patients were most likely to
develop post-traumatic seizures remained unclear.

This monograph reports studies directed to answering Symonds'
challenging questions and redressing the situation alluded to by Garland. It
seemed likely that the best chance of discovering something more definite
about the natural history of traumatic epilepsy would be for one person to
study a sufficiently large number of cases and to be ruthless in excluding
all those on whom only uncertain or inadequate details were available.

The questions demanding an answer are these. How often does epilepsy
occur in the acute stage of a head injury, and what is its significance, as far
as the present and the future are concerned? What is the incidence of late
epilepsy and what is its nature and course? Are there any features of the

1

acute stage of a head injury which enable some prediction to be made of the likelihood of fits developing later? Such questions are of interest not only to doctors responsible for treating and advising patients, but to the judge who often has to decide, when awarding damages, whether epilepsy is likely to develop subsequent to a particular injury; and if it does occur, or already has done, how likely it is to persist and to constitute a disability?

Categorical answers to this question are often demanded from medical men by lawyers. This may account for the tendency of doctors to make the kind of dogmatic statement based on flimsy evidence which characterises the literature on traumatic epilepsy. There is as little room for honest agnosticism in the courts as there is for dishonest dogmatism in academic medicine. It is not long before a tentative assertion made in the first few minutes in the witness box is puffed up by gentle persuasion and mild flattery until even the humblest doctor is able to see it as a didactic statement by an eminent authority. It is not surprising that these opinions soon appear in medical journals and eventually get written into one textbook and copied by others. The clarity and assurance of these is such, however, that they appeal to the pragmatic practitioner more concerned with *an* answer than with *the* answer to a question.

This is a clinical study, directed at determining facts about the frequency and nature of epilepsy after different kinds of injury. No pathological material has been examined nor is the literature of the pathology discussed. It was not originally intended to give an account of the EEG findings because they were so incomplete; but this investigation is so often invoked in discussions on traumatic epilepsy that a brief report has been included of the principal abnormalities found in the patients studied.

This is intended to be a factual report about the natural history of traumatic epilepsy. Recommendations about treatment are made only in the most general terms, because references to drugs are apt soon to be outdated. The aim is to provide information on which to decide whether to offer treatment and if so how long it should be continued, and by which its efficacy might be judged. Similarly there is little discussion or speculation about the causes and origins of epilepsy after trauma, which would have to take account of many other sources of information, both clinical and experimental, which are not strictly relevant to the present studies. But it is hoped that anyone putting forward hypotheses to explain traumatic epilepsy would consider it necessary to take account of the data presented here.

Chapter 2

THE LITERATURE

"The worst of Warburton is, that he has a rage for saying something, when there's nothing to be said."

Samuel Johnson (1758)

There is both an abundance and a scarcity of writings on traumatic epilepsy. Trivial references abound in the form of asides in papers on epilepsy, and after-thoughts in papers on head injuries. Few studies have been directed specifically to traumatic epilepsy, and of these even fewer report a sufficient number of adequately documented cases for the conclusions to be taken as serious contributions to existing knowledge. As long ago as 1904 a Hunterian lecturer was pleading that the literature on traumatic epilepsy was almost more than one man could deal with. A lot of ink has flowed since then. If a complete account were to be given even of the English language writings on this subject a chapter would result which would be as tedious as it would be confusing. What makes the reading of the literature so frustrating, and would render a slavish recounting of it fruitless, is the difficulty of judging from most papers what kind of injuries the patients under discussion had suffered, how many had been followed up and for how long, and what criteria had determined the diagnosis of traumatic epilepsy. That, rather than the sheer bulk of the literature, is my defence for giving only a restricted account of the literature. Moreover there is no need to trace the evolution of technical developments to put the present study into perspective, because it depends only on the timeless equipment of accurate clinical observation adequately recorded.

Four out of five publications which were read in the original, including some well-known accounts, have been omitted, usually because the definitions were not clear enough to draw useful conclusions from the data presented. Most often no distinction was made between missile and non-missile injuries in series presumed to be made up of both. The present study is concerned only with one type of injury, and indeed seeks to identify differences which depend on the type of injury; comparisons with mixed series are therefore of limited relevance.

The year before the first edition of this monograph a medico-legal text claimed that no authentic statistics existed for the frequency of epilepsy after closed head injury (Worcester-Drought, 1961). This is not quite fair

3

to the memory of the late Gilbert Phillips whose posthumously published study of traumatic epilepsy after closed injuries in soldiers was a real attempt to investigate a large series in a critical fashion (Phillips, 1954). Indeed this paper was the point of departure for the present work; and as the same punch card he devised has been used many of the groupings of cases are the same as his. The limitations of his work were the selected population (servicemen only) and the relatively short period of follow-up. What is true is that no report so far has been able to base conclusions on statistical tests of probability, because no series has been large enough for statistical significance to be attained in the small sub-groups representing the many factors which may influence the development of this complication and determine the course it may take. Since this monograph was first published there have been a number of reports, some perhaps prompted by it, and these are now included in the brief account of the literature which appears at the beginning of each section.

Chapter 3

DEFINITION OF A HEAD INJURY

"General terms are made use of, by which no precise idea is conveyed, and the surgeon not clear in his own conception of the nature of the disease is at a loss to account for it to others."

Percival Pott (1759)

That the concept of what constitutes a head injury should need definition is less obvious than the need to recognise the type and severity of the injury. But any assessment of the incidence of epilepsy after injury is meaningless unless the minimal criteria taken to constitute a head injury are declared.

What matters in a head injury is damage to the brain, either on impact or subsequently due to processes initiated by that impact. Fatal brain damage can occur without fracture of the skull or any blemish on the scalp, but lacerations and fractures are evidence of local violence and the likelihood of underlying brain damage. Although Munro (1938) stated that "no significant cerebral injury occurs without some degree of unconsciousness", Denny-Brown (1941) defined a head injury as "such injury to the skull as might directly or indirectly damage the brain, even when there is no unconsciousness (i.e. no concussion)". As long ago as 1921, Turner and Eden had stated that cortical contusion could occur without any amnesia; indeed it is well recognised that local contusion and even laceration of the cortex frequently occurs under a compound depressed fracture in patients who have never been unconscious (Miller and Jennett, 1968; Jennett and Miller, 1972). Clearly brain damage need not cause altered consciousness; but loss of consciousness or even brief amnesia after injury always implies brain damage.

The term "concussion" enjoys no universally accepted definition, but it is so widely used that some attempt must be made to come to terms with it. In Trotter's original description in 1924, concussion referred to the brief period of altered consciousness after mild injuries which, although rapidly recovered from, was always followed by amnesia for the actual moment of the accident. Although many would still agree with this usage, Symonds (1962) has recently suggested that unconsciousness lasting hours or even days after an injury, but not associated with focal signs or obvious complications, should be regarded as prolonged concussion because the

5

difference in brain damage is of degree rather than of kind. There may be reluctance to accept such a radical change in the concept of concussion but it would now be generally agreed that even the mildest "concussion" produces permanent neurological damage of some degree. And two components of the original definition, that concussion implied an absence of structural damage and also freedom of sequelae, would certainly now be rejected.

No one criterion will adequately define head injury or brain damage, but for the practical purpose of defining a population of head injuries it seemed best to consider all patients admitted to hospital. This includes injuries of widely varying severity, yet excludes the many cases about which there is doubt even about whether a head injury was sustained at all. Most hospitals in developed countries adopt a policy of admitting all patients with a history of unconsciousness after injury, or with amnesia for the accident, as well as those with a skull fracture — whether or not associated with altered consciousness. Such a policy results in the admission to hospital of many patients with mild injuries which are therefore included. It is important to avoid the fallacy of cyclical definition — assuming *ab initio* that trivial injuries cannot cause epilepsy and by excluding all injuries of less than a given severity from the study ensuring that only the more severe injuries will ever be accepted as causing epilepsy. Many of the widespread discrepancies between different reports about epilepsy after non-missile injury can be traced to differences in the population analysed. Bowers (1921) stated that injury may occasion epilepsy without any visible lesion of the brain and Symonds (1935) said epilepsy could follow an injury without concussion. Yet Muskens (1928) held that traumatic epilepsy should not be diagnosed unless there was a fracture, whilst Penfield (1954) insisted that the injury must in some way affect the grey matter (but he did not indicate how to detect such an affection).

Severity of Injury

With such a wide range of injuries to be considered it is essential to be able to compare the severity of different cases. Yet few authors in their papers, or clinicians in their case notes, enlighten their readers on the evidence by which they judge one injury to be more severe than another and paradoxical statements emerge such as "had a severe head injury", "no fracture, no loss of consciousness". With missile injuries and non-missile depressed fractures the degree of local damage may best be judged by the extent and depth of the wound, and there may also be focal neurological signs which reflect local brain damage. But the severity of the diffuse brain damage which results from the acceleration/deceleration forces generated by blunt trauma (and which may also accompany local damage in penetrating injuries) is best judged by the duration of the post-traumatic amnesia (PTA). It is more than 40 years since Ritchie Russell (1932), then a young intern in Edinburgh, proposed that the lapse of time between the injury and the return of continuous memory might be a useful indication of the severity of injury. Since then evidence has steadily accumulated (Symonds and Russell, 1943; Smith and Russell, 1961; Lishman, 1962) to support the view that PTA provides the best available guide to the severity of diffuse brain injury.

A convenience of using the PTA as a measure of severity is that it can be assessed without reference to clinical notes or to the evidence of witnesses, by asking the patient how long it was before he became aware of his surroundings. It is usually possible to assess this within broad limits, even months or years after the injury; the categories proposed by Russell remain appropriate (nil, less than an hour, 1-24 hours, 1-7 days and more than a week). For most analyses in this study only two categories are used, more or less than 24 hours, because it is almost always possible to allocate patients to one of these categories with confidence. When determining the PTA it is well to remember that the capacity of the brain to store day to day memories is one of the last functions to return after diffuse brain damage. Patients are frequently regarded as having regained consciousness, as judged by their beginning to speak, to recognise relatives, to feed themselves, yet subsequent inquiry reveals that they have no memory of the early part of this period of recovery. Sometimes there may be islands of memory, especially when PTA has lasted only a day or so; the patient remembers fragments of an ambulance journey, or of being X-rayed or of having stitches put in his head. In assessing PTA it is the return of continuous memory which counts, and it is important that this should be the patient's own account, not that of relatives who are likely to report a much shorter period of "unconsciousness" because they will usually have judged this to have ended when the patient began to speak. Sometimes the patient will report this period also, because his family have told him that he was in coma for only a few hours or a certain number of days, although his own experience was that it was much longer before he "woke up". Retrospective assessment of PTA has been emphasised because in the context of studying traumatic epilepsy and in the clinical practice of predicting the risk of epilepsy, that is usually how it has to be done. When PTA lasts several days its duration has been found to correspond closely with the period of disorientation, and its end with the return of awareness of time and place; experienced staff seeing the patient every day in the acute stage seldom have much doubt about when the patient "comes out of PTA".

Amnesia may of course be simulated. Certain sections of the community which are prone to accidents know that to profess it may be advantageous, not only because it may be taken as evidence of a head injury but because it also absolves the victim from having to give any account of the circumstances surrounding the accident. Of 65 cases of epilepsy seeking litigation in the United States on account of a preceding head injury alleged to have caused the fits, 12 were found never to have suffered the head injury they claimed, and 28 had materially exaggerated the severity of their injury (Hyslop, 1950). Retrograde amnesia, loss of memory for events prior to the head injury, shows a very poor correlation with the severity of that injury; after relatively mild injuries patients may profess loss of memory for hours, weeks or even months prior to the injury. This amnesia commonly contracts with time, whereas the post-traumatic amnesia is very stable and seems not to be influenced by psychological factors.

Type of Injury

Head injuries are commonly classified according to the mechanism by which they are caused. In civilian life most injuries are blunt, at least in Britain. The head strikes a blunt object, usually the road, producing abrupt deceleration which results in diffuse brain damage; such injuries may result in anterior fossa fractures into the air sinuses or in compound vault fractures, and it is inappropiate to term them "closed" head injuries although this is often done to distinguish them from penetrating gunshot wounds. Low velocity penetrating injuries occur due to assault (and sometimes accidents) involving sharp objects such as scissors, sticks, knives, knitting needles and the like. These differ from missile injuries in that high velocity objects on entering the skull tend to produce more extensive damage; low velocity injuries are frequently under-estimated until complications develop and the patient may not even report for medical attention (Jennett and Miller, 1972). It is clearly unsatisfactory to classify injuries into civilian and military, because in some countries civilians inflict many missile injuries on each other, whilst the military sustain many blunt injuries in the course of their duty. It seems that the most satisfactory classification is missle and non-missile, and it is more appropriate to regard this study as pertaining to non-missile injuries than to blunt injuries, which was the term used in the title of the first edition.

Chapter 4

DEFINITION OF EPILEPSY

"A fit, is a fit, is a fit."
Professor E. B. Shaw of San Francisco
(after Gertrude Stein)

Until fairly recently the term "epilepsy" was largely confined to general and focal convulsions, although as long ago as 1903 Gowers had explored what he called the "borderlands of epilepsy". Certainly it is to these two forms that most references are made in connection with traumatic epilepsy. The recent recognition of the frequency and variety of temporal lobe seizures has led to the acceptance of many phenomena as epileptic which had hitherto been ascribed to other causes. In the context of a florid post-concussional syndrome it is easy to imagine how automatisms and episodic anomalies of behaviour might be attributed to a psychological mechanism, and momentary absences confused with positional vertigo. Denny-Brown (1943) reported the association of "quasi-fugal" states with traumatic epilepsy as more common than could be expected from coincidence, and it seems likely that he was in fact describing temporal lobe seizures. Vitale *et al.* (1953) actually reported forty cases of temporal lobe epilepsy thought to be traumatic in origin.

No generally accepted classification of seizures exists. This renders recording arbitrary, discussion difficult and comparisons of reported series almost impossible. The most that can be done is to define terms, apply them rigidly to the whole group, and explain those particulars in which the scheme differs from those most frequently met with in other reports.

Penfield's distinction (1954) between focal and local attacks is apposite, especially as we are anxious to discern, if we can, any evidence for the anatomical origin of the seizures. He maintained that an attack should be regarded as *focal* if if had a demonstrable origin in an area of the grey matter of one cerebral hemisphere, no matter how widely the seizure activity might ultimately spread. He did not cite how such an origin was to be determined, but it seems clear from the context that it is from the nature of the clinical onset of the fit that the distinction is to be made. He classified focal attacks as motor, sensory, psychical and automatisms. With careful documentation, talking with relatives and prolonged observation more and more patients come into this group, and the once large group of generalized convulsions is depleted *pari passu.*

9

This distinction between focal and non-focal attacks has been adopted as the basis of classifying attacks in the present study. Many patients had more than one type of attack, but if any of these betrayed a focal origin then that patient was regarded as having focal attacks.

Whilst every effort was made to detect a focal origin in these cases there are doubtless some patients who are in the non-focal group not because there was impeccable evidence that there was no focality about the onset, but simply because there was insufficient evidence of focal features. That a person is found convulsing, incontinent and with a bitten tongue is sufficient evidence of epilepsy; it may never be possible to document the early events of a seizure. So the focal group here, as almost certainly in all other series, represents the minimum number of patients belonging in it.

The different types of seizures recognised were as follows:

Non-focal

1. Grand mal
2. Akinetic (general)
3. "Petit mal"

Focal

1. Focal motor
2. Focal sensory
3. Focal onset but generalising
4. Focal temporal

Whilst most of these terms are self-explanatory some require further definition.

Akinetic (general) attacks consisted of a period of unconsciousness, usually lasting from 5 to 30 minutes, during which the patient was inert and limp but without convulsions. This seems preferable to using the term minor grand mal.

"Petit mal" demands some comment because it may be confused with temporal lobe seizures. It is a term confined by some workers to attacks occurring many times a day in children, and by many others to such attacks only if accompanied by a specific spike and wave EEG record. No case satisfying these definitions was met with in the present study. But the term is still widely used for momentary lapses without evidence of temporal lobe involvement and it is difficult to avoid its use. Renfrew *et al.* (1957) retain it in their very logical classification, and their definition has been accepted here. This is a mental blank of short duration (less than 30 seconds), with no premonition of it and unaccompanied by any automatic behaviour except minimal fumbling of the hands. This can closely resemble minor temporal lobe seizures without automatisms of a definitely recognisable kind in which, however, the blank period often lasts for a few minutes and the patient may sit down, stare, perhaps mumble or fumble a little but neither falls nor indulges in sufficiently organised activity to earn the title of automatism. To distinguish between the two is not easy, and as in other cases dubious cases will end up in the non-focal group, classified as petit mal, when perhaps they should have been classified as temporal lobe fits.

Two types of attack have not been accepted as epileptic at all, although some authors have claimed that this is their nature.

Penfield included in his motor group *"tonic mesencephalic attacks"*. It is not appropriate to discuss whether or not these spasmodic outbursts of nervous activity in the midbrain should be regarded as epileptic. Suffice it to say that they are common in the early phases of severe head injuries, under the label of decerebrate attacks, that they seem never to have been admitted for discussion as a form of traumatic epilepsy and that they are similarly excluded here.

More controversial are the *vertiginous episodes* so common in the early months after a closed head injury. Next to headache they form the principal complaint of patients with the so-called post-concussive syndrome. In discussing 1,657 cases of vertigo of peripheral origin Cawthorne (1952) cites head injury as the commonest cause after Ménière's disease. Some of these patients may suffer from central vestibular damage, for Groat *et al.* (1945) found that in experimentally concussed animals the maximal cellular changes were in the lateral vestibular nucleus. The vertigo is often positional, which suggests that it is due to a peripheral disorder.

Nonetheless several authors with extensive personal experience of these patients have expressed the view that postural vertigo may suffer a transition into frank epilepsy. To quote Symonds (1935), "if the early minor attacks of momentary cessation of clear awareness with a tendency to fall are adequately treated they are less likely to develop into frank epilepsy". In fact these attacks are notoriously resistant to treatment; phenobarbitone rarely controls them, and if there is some improvement it is as likely to be because this drug acts as a labyrinthine sedative as to be due to its anticonvulsant properties.

There are certainly attacks in which it is difficult to determine whether the tendency to fall is due to transitory clouding of consciousness, but most patients with these vertiginous episodes give a good account of them. There is the sudden sensation of movement, frequently precipitated by rapid head movements or stooping down, and very short-lived. The attacks frequently outlive other symptoms and some patients, though able to return to work, have to change, on account of vertigo, from an occupation which involves awkward head movements.

Vertiginous disorders following closed head injuries are so common, so constantly related to posture and they so constantly disperse with time that it is difficult to discern any relationship between them and subsequent epilepsy. Their very frequency makes it inevitable that they will have been the concern at one time of a number of patients who later develop fits. If the rarity of such attacks apart from head injury is recalled, together with the frequency in many other conditions of epilepsy of various kinds, the case for regarding them as related to epilepsy seems insupportable.

The decision as to whether or not epilepsy had occurred was always made on clinical evidence, and never on the basis of the EEG. Dubious attacks were always rejected.

Chapter 5

DEFINITION OF TRAUMATIC EPILEPSY

"I never 'ad this 'ere epilepsy afore I 'it me 'ead" – a patient.
"Res ipse loquator" – his lawyer.

Having defined both trauma and epilepsy it remains to indicate when the one is to be regarded as causally related to the other. Any criteria proposed must be arbitary, for it is seldom that the relationship can be more than presumptive. When appropriate focal attacks follow local penetrating injuries such as a depressed fracture, there will be little doubt about the connection. Implication of a head injury as the cause of epileptic attacks must also hinge on excluding other causes of epilepsy. In the opinion of some a fairly close relationship in time is required but this adds nothing to the precision of the definition. There are well-documented cases beginning 30-40 years after missile injuries, closely related to the scar. It is clearly unjustifiable to exclude a fit as due to trauma because of the time interval alone, although this is frequently and authoritatively proposed.

The demand for the exclusion of other possible causes for a fit occurring after an injury is a reasonable one, but hard to satisfy. In the young, idiopathic epilepsy, and in the elderly, cerebral arteriosclerosis are common but neither is susceptible of precise diagnosis in many cases. Angiomas and cerebral tumours may cause fits for years before local neurological defects, increased pressure or subarachnoid haemorrhage draw attention to the true state of affairs, and these conditions may occasionally elude detection even by angiography and air encephalography. It is no surprise therefore to read Sheehan's account (1958) of a man in receipt of a pension for traumatic epilepsy developing a cerebral tumour which had almost certainly accounted for his fits all along.

However, such a course is unusual, and most patients with symptomatic epilepsy will show some sign of the underlying condition within a year or two of the appearance of epilepsy. Therefore a follow-up for some time after the first fit will guard against the inclusion of patients with other organic diseases and a great many of the patients in the present study were in fact followed for several years after the onset of epilepsy. Moreover as the neurosurgical units concerned enjoyed virtual geographical monopolies during the time that these cases were being collected there was a great likelihood that any patient referred with epilepsy and subsequently developing further signs of brain damage would have been referred back to that clinic. Later development of tumour or other disease can therefore be presumed unlikely even in those not actively followed up.

It has been asserted that one or two fits do not warrant the diagnosis of epilepsy, which should be restricted to the description of established, continuing or recurring fits. The practice of other authors in accepting one fit as sufficient evidence for the diagnosis of post-traumatic epilepsy has been adopted here (Russell and Whitty, 1952; Phillips, 1954). That some patients suffer only one or very few attacks, even after prolonged follow-up, is acknowledged but it seems unhelpful, and indeed untruthful, to regard those with fewer than a certain number of fits as not having suffered from epilepsy.

A distinction is made throughout this work between early and late epilepsy, fits in the first week after injury being designated early. The case for recognising epilepsy in the first week as a separate entity depends on evidence from the present study, and this appears in Chapter 8, where the literature is also discussed. Patients who have a fit in the first week and who subsequently have one or more fits after this period are regarded as suffering from both early and late epilepsy.

Chapter 6

PATIENTS STUDIED AND METHODS USED

To elucidate this problem there had to be large enough numbers for patterns of relationships to be revealed; but a certain minimum amount of verifiable information had to be available about every case, even if this entailed a sacrifice of numbers. The demand for large numbers, together with the time lapses which form an essential part of such a study, precluded the possibility of collecting a personal series, and made inevitable some dependence on the written records of others. The best that could be done to ensure some degree of consistency in such circumstances was for one person alone to make all the assessments from the original case notes, and this I myself did.

Two different types of patient can be studied, the information in each case being subject to different sources of error. One consists of the recently injured person, observed at the time of his initial hospital admission and subsequently followed up. Details about the injury are usually available and information about the incidence and nature of early fits is likely to be reliable. But keeping in touch with large numbers of such patients, expecially those who have had only mild injuries, for long enough to observe not only the development of late epilepsy but the course of this complication, presents problems. Details about late epilepsy are more easily ascertained from patients who present with epilepsy and who are found to have suffered from a head injury in the past. Many of these are first seen a long time after injury when it may be difficult to discover full details about the original injury; even when the original notes can be found the quantity and quality of information they contain is often disappointing. The advantages enjoyed by those who have studied military cases is emphasised by this experience. During the World War II it became customary in Britain, largely due to the example and leadership of Sir Hugh Cairns, to make full notes about head injured men even in advanced areas, and these valuable documents were available for later study; similar advantageous circumstances have led to useful data from the Korean conflict, and more recently from Vietnam.

Sources of Cases

Since the beginning of this study 17 years ago several different patient populations have been studied and the chronological sequence of this aggregation of patients should be understood.

15

The Oxford 1,000 Series

The study began with the analysis of the occurrence of epilepsy in 1,000 consecutive head injuries admitted to the Radcliffe Infirmary in Oxford between 1948 and 1952. This indicated the importance of distinguishing between *early* epilepsy (first week after injury) and *late* epilepsy. The sample of 275 patients followed up for 4 years or more identified three factors as predominant in predisposing to late epilepsy — namely early epilepsy, depressed fracture and acute intracranial haematoma (evacuation within 14 days of injury) (Jennett and Lewin, 1960).

The importance of this series lies in its being composed of consecutive cases of non-missile head injury admitted to a single hospital, which was the only one taking in head injuries for many miles around. Among them were many cases of mild injury, because the criterion for admission in doubtful cases was evidence of cerebral concussion as judged by a period of amnesia, even if brief. The casualty officers concerned with the admission were trained to seek for evidence of this with the result that many mild cases were taken into hospital who might have been sent home by other institutions. Thus less than 20% were amnesic for more than 24 hours and 58% had a PTA of less than an hour; less than half had a fractured skull. Although there were some cases transferred from outlying hospitals with major injuries or suspected complications it is felt that this series as a whole represents as nearly ùnselected a group of hospital head injuries as is ever likely to be available for study. Those patients who had had previous epilepsy were excluded, leaving 986 injuries for analysis. Not all previous authors make this obviously important adjustment; Phillips (1954) mentions that of 31 patients in his unselected series who developed epilepsy, 4 (13%) had had previous attacks. Previous epilepsy may not be declared even if inquiries are made, but that is an imponderable in every series.

Additional Cases for the First Edition

The next stage was to gather more patients with early epilepsy, or depressed fracture or haematoma; the analysis of this larger series confirmed that these three factors did indeed contribute significantly to the risk of late epilepsy. However, complex inter-relationships began to emerge between these and other factors, but there were still too few patients available for the probability of epilepsy in some of the smaller subgroups to be calculated. Clearly, even more cases were required to provide a statistically sound basis for making predictions in individual patients as distinct from populations.

Glasgow and Rotterdam Cases

Moving to Glasgow in 1963 gave me the opportunity to collect many more cases, this time from a neurosurgical unit to which head injuries were secondarily referred by general hospitals to which they had first been admitted. Although such cases were selected, they included almost all patients in the district with the conditions with which this study was now concerned — early epilepsy, depressed fracture, and haematoma. As a diversion from the epilepsy study, the whole range of complications following depressed fracture was investigated (Miller and Jennett, 1968). This in turn led Dr. Braakman of Rotterdam to compare a series of depressed fractures in his clinic with the Glasgow series, and to report that the two were remarkably similar (Braakman, 1972). As he used a similar method of analysis, the Rotterdam cases were suitable for the epilepsy study, and he kindly agreed to their being added to the present series. There are now over 1,000 patients with depressed fracture in the study and 420 with acute intracranial haematoma. There are 436 with early epilepsy and 481 with late epilepsy; as 90 patients had both early and late epilepsy, there are 802 patients with traumatic epilepsy of one kind or another (6/1).

6/1   *Accumulation of cases in present study*

	Oxford 1000 series (1960)	First edition (1962)	Second edition (1974)
Total traumatic epilepsy	64	381	827
Total early epilepsy	46	139	436
Total late epilepsy	28	282	481
Both early and late epilepsy	10	40	90
Depressed fracture	74	134	1005
Acute IC haematoma	58	79	420

Comparison Between Cases from Different Sources

The additional cases were therefore compared with corresponding cases in the Oxford 1,000 series in respect of certain features; there proved to be no significant difference (6/2, 6/3, 6/4). For depressed fractures a close resemblance was shown between those collected from three different cities (Fig. 1).

6/2   *Features of early epilepsy patients in Oxford 1000 series and in additional cases*

Feature	Oxford 1000 46		Additional 371		P
<5 years	7	15%	71	19%	NS
>16 years	35	76%	206	56%	<0.01
PTA >24 hours	$^{18}/_{38}$	47%	$^{141}/_{346}$	41%	NS
Depressed fracture	9	20%	87	23%	NS
IC haematoma	13	28%	99	27%	NS
No depressed fracture or haematoma	24	52%	185	50%	NS

The striking similarity found between the series of patients assembled from sources which differed considerably, both in socio-economic terms and in hospital admission arrangements, suggests that the patients studied are indeed reasonably representative samples of the universe of patients suffering from these particular types of injury.

Follow-up Series

To determine the incidence of late epilepsy calls for the prolonged follow-up of large numbers of unselected injuries. This is difficult to do. The problem is the dubious wisdom and propriety of demanding repeated attendance at hospital, or even the answering of questionnaires, by relatively mildly injured patients. The litigious leanings of this group of patients towards the party whom they hold to blame for their accident is well known, and the sooner their recovery can be emphasised by unconditional discharge from hospital the more likely they are to complete and maintain this recovery. Almost inevitably therefore an error enters into assessments of incidence of late epilepsy, due to the more efficient following of the more severely injured patients. In that the follow-up in this study has concentrated on high risk groups the present series is not free from this bias, although this has been allowed for when calculating overall incidence, by taking account of the distribution of these types of injury in the series of unselected injuries from Oxford (p. 95). The one year follow-up rates achieved for the three main groups are indicated in 6/5, 6/6, 6/7.

6/3   *Features of depressed fracture patients in Oxford 1000 series and in additional cases*

Feature	Oxford 1000 74		Additional 893		P
< 5 years	11	15%	133	15%	NS
> 16 years	49	66%	439	50%	< 0.01
PTA > 24 hours	$^{17}/_{63}$	27%	$^{213}/_{864}$	25%	NS
Dura torn	$^{30}/_{60}$	50%	$^{399}/_{780}$	50%	NS
Early epilepsy	9	12%	87	10%	NS

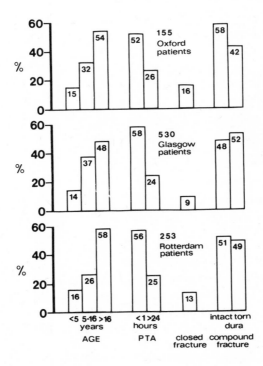

Fig. 1. Characteristics of depressed fractures from three cities.

6/4   *Features of haematoma patients in Oxford 1000 series and in additional cases*

Feature	Oxford 1000 58		Additional 362		P
< 16 years	9	16%	59	16%	NS
Extradural	23	40%	123	34%	NS
PTA > 24 hours	$^{24}/_{42}$	57%	$^{168}/_{346}$	49%	NS
Early epilepsy	13	23%	99	27%	NS

6/5   *Features of original early epilepsy series and of those followed*

Feature	Original 417		Followed up 238		P
< 5 years	78	19%	42	18%	NS
> 16 years	241	58%	120	50%	NS
PTA > 24 hours	$^{146}/_{366}$	40%	$^{94}/_{234}$	40%	NS
Focal signs	106	25%	69	29%	NS
Depressed fracture	98	24%	81	34%	NS
Intracranial haematoma	112	27%	35	15%	<0.001
No depressed fracture or haematoma	209	50%	124	52%	NS

Each series successfully followed up was compared with the original population for that type of injury, to verify that there was no important difference; in the event the correspondence was close (6/6, 6/7, 6/8). The relative consistency of the epilepsy incidence as the number of patients has increased over the years (Fig. 2) suggests that the methods used to collect cases and to detect this complication are free from serious bias reflecting different local circumstances, or changing attitudes or practices during the years spanned by this study.

No further information has been collected since the first edition about the incidence of late epilepsy in head injuries who do *not* have one of the

6/6 *Features of original depressed fracture series and of those followed*

	Original 947		Followed up 693		P
<5 years	138	15%	109	16%	NS
>16 years	488	51%	348	50%	NS
PTA > 24 hours	$230/927$	25%	$168/688$	24%	NS
Focal signs	192	20%	148	21%	NS
Early epilepsy	96	10%	81	12%	NS

6/7 *Features of original haematoma series and of those followed*

Feature	Original 420		Followed up 128		P
<5 years	28	7%	9	7%	NS
>16 years	352	84%	100	78%	NS
PTA > 24 hours	$210/382$	55%	$79/126$	63%	NS
Extradural	146	35%	59	48%	NS
Focal signs	175	42%	73	57%	<0.01
Early epilepsy	112	27%	35	27%	NS

6/8 *Incidence of LATE epilepsy in actual and extrapolated follow-up series* without *certain features of injury*

	No depressed fracture		No early epilepsy		No haematoma	
In Oxford follow-up	$17/223$	8%	$18/240$	8%	$18/240$	8%
In Oxford 1000 by extrapolation	$27/832$	3%	$29/868$	3%	$27/854$	3%

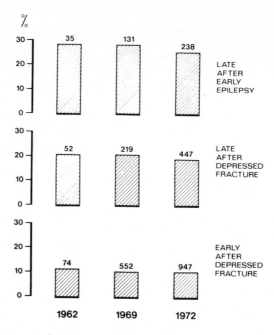

Fig. 2. Epilepsy rates during accumulation of series, showing how constant these have been.

three predisposing factors. The total series of patients now in the study contains an undue proportion of those with a high risk of epilepsy. When a comparison is sought between patients with and without, say, depressed fracture, it would be misleading to regard the rest of the present series as representative of unselected injuries without depressed fracture. Most comparisons therefore depend on the sample of the original Oxford series which was followed up, but even that sample was somewhat biased with high risk cases, in spite of the deliberate tracing of the first consecutive 100 injuries with less than 1 hour's amnesia and uncomplicated by early epilepsy, depressed fracture or haematoma. By extrapolation from those actually followed up to the 1,000 series, taking account of the frequency with which different types of injury occurred within that series, it has been possible to estimate the incidence of late epilepsy for head injuries without early epilepsy, or without depressed fracture, or without acute haematoma (6/8). This figure is naturally lower than that for those which were actually followed, but it is the truest estimate; the figure reached by this means for injuries without early epilepsy corresponds closely to that for a followed series published by Stowsand and Bues (1970). Lack of data prevented such an extrapolated estimate being made for sub-groups which take account of factors other than the three dominant ones; consequently the epilepsy rate in the "factor absent" line of these tables is likely to be somewhat higher than it would be in an unselected series. A further consequence of this is that the epileptogenic influence of the factors being explored in these sub-groups tends to be minimised.

Statistics and Presentation

The main purpose of this study has been to explore the influence of various factors on the incidence and character of early and late epilepsy. Statisticians consulted at various stages in the evolution of the project have all given the same advice, that the best way to achieve this objective was to keep the analysis at the simple level of 2 x 2 tables. Although combinations of factors have been considered, these have likewise been reduced to a series of 2 x 2 tables. For all these the statistical significance has been tested using the chi^2 probability test, using Yates' correction for a discontinuous series. When P = >0.05 the difference is recorded as "not significant (NS)". All percentages have been rounded to the nearest whole number, 0.5 being rounded up.

An Apology

The literary shorthand of referring to patients with, for example, depressed fracture or haematoma as so many "depressed fractures" or "haematomas" has occasionally been resorted to by way of preventing the text and tables becoming unduly turgid and repetitive. Perhaps because it is recognised, and resorted to with good intentions, this solecism may be forgiven.

Chapter 7

HEAD INJURIES IN PATIENTS WITH PREVIOUS EPILEPSY

Whilst there were not sufficient patients with previous epilepsy who were studied following head injury for any formal analysis to be possible, it is interesting to see what did happen to these few patients, who are excluded from all subsequent analyses.

In the 1,000 series there were 14 with a known epileptic history. This is higher than the incidence in the population at large (commonly quoted as 0.5%), which is doubtless due to the liability of epileptics to sustain head injuries during their attacks. It is possible that there are other undeclared epileptics in this series in spite of every attempt to exclude them, for it is not uncommon for previous fits to be denied when the question of litigation arises. Indeed in two patients the history of epilepsy was only discovered by a circuitous route after this investigation had been underway for some time, and after they had both been regarded as *bona fide* traumatic epileptics.

The severity of the injuries suffered by these 14 patients, as judged by the PTA, corresponded closely to that for the 1,000 as a whole. There was only one who had a fit in the first week after injury. During the period of follow-up six had further fits, in all cases following the pattern characteristic of that particular patient's epilepsy before injury.

During the collection of further cases of early epilepsy after injury 8 more patients were encountered making 9 in all who were excluded from the study because they were known to have had at least one fit previous to the injury. There were 4 who had had only occasional fits, two of them having had none for over 14 years before the injury; the other two were adults who had had seizures only in infancy. They were not therefore established epileptics, in the ordinary sense of the term. One of them had a series of generalised attacks immediately after injury, but had no further attacks during the succeeding 10 years; this is in line with the behaviour of all other patients who had attacks immediately after injury, in that late epilepsy did not develop. It differs in that there was a series of attacks, whilst immediate epilepsy in those who had not had previous fits was always limited to a single seizure. Two of these 4 patients whose pre-traumatic epilepsy had been dormant for years did suffer fits again

24

later, 6 months and 2 years after the injury, and continued to suffer from frequent epilepsy thereafter.

The 4 with more persistent epilepsy had all had a year's freedom from attacks immediately preceding the injury which was complicated by an early fit. Of these, two had early traumatic fits similar in pattern to their usual attacks, but two who normally experienced generalised fits had focal motor attacks during the early stages after injury; the one of these who was followed up reverted to his normal pattern of epilepsy after the acute post-traumatic phase.

Chapter 8

THE IDENTITY OF EARLY EPILEPSY

Epilepsy occurring soon after injury is treated separately by many authors, as though to imply that the cause or the course of fits at this time may be different from epilepsy developing later.

Fits in the first month and not repeated later were set on one side by Russell and Whitty (1952), whilst Phillips (1954) and Whitty (1947) each recognised fits within two weeks of injury as a separate category. Both Elvidge (1949) and Mock (1950) suggested that early fits should be sub-divided into immediate, delayed and convalescent. Evans (1962) found no fits between the 18th day after injury and the fourth week, so that defining early epilepsy as within 18 days of injury was in fact expressing the seizure rate for the first month after injury.

Discussing basic mechanisms Caveness (1964) separated influences acting at the moment of impact, within minutes or hours, within hours or days and within the first few weeks. More simply Walker (1969), also concerned with pathogenesis, distinguished only the *immediate* fit, *early* convulsions (few hours or days after injury) and *late* epilepsy (weeks or months after injury). Denny-Brown (1943) expressed concern that patients with early fits might be labelled as cases of traumatic epilepsy, which he thought unjustified, and he suggested the term "immediate epilepsy". However, this term is more usually applied, both in the literature and in this book, for the small group of early fits which occur within the first few moments after injury, because these proved to have certain features in common. To judge from the literature there is very little danger of patients with epilepsy being labelled epileptic — more often they are dismissed altogether from discussions of traumatic epilepsy. For example, Glaser and Schafer (1945) wrote, "any case in which epileptic seizures of a generalised type develop after a minor injury within the period of several weeks is immediately excluded from the post-traumatic group". It will be shown that this cavalier gesture ignores the facts of the case.

Clearly no consensus has emerged about how early is early, and authors have variously referred to epilepsy within one, two, three and four weeks of injury as "early", without defending their choice of time interval, which appears to have been arbitrary. Indeed Whitty (1947) pointed out that early fits tend to occur "when widespread delayed effects of injury are at a

26

maximum" and he suggested that a physiological rather than a strictly temporal definition should be utilised in defining this type of epilepsy. However, physiological states are not as readily assessed as the passage of time and the present study provides evidence in support of a temporal definition, the end of the first week proving to be a natural watershed.

The Present Series

In the closely observed Oxford injuries there were 46 patients with epilepsy during the first week and only one patient had his first fit between the end of the first week and the eleventh week after injury (Jennett and Lewin, 1960). This led us, at that time, to define *early* epilepsy as that occurring within a week of injury. With subsequent enlargement of the population studied some patients have been encountered in whom the first fit did occur in the first few weeks following the first week. Questions then arise as to whether these are delayed "early" fits, or are premature "late" fits – and whether the end of the first week does in fact form a true watershed? The answers depend on four separate strands of evidence – the time after injury of the first fit, the type of fit suffered, the risk of epilepsy recurring in the future, and the factors which influence the incidence of epilepsy at different intervals after injury. The data which indicates, in respect of each of these aspects of traumatic epilepsy, that the first week is in fact different will now be presented.

Time of First Fit within 2 Months of Injury

In 414 patients with epilepsy beginning within 8 weeks of injury the time of the first fit was recorded; if a patient had a fit in the first week and again, at say 4 weeks, only the first fit was recorded. Note that this is at variance with all subsequent analyses in this book, where such a patient would be regarded as having both early and late epilepsy. About half of these patients were from Oxford and the rest from Glasgow, which provided the opportunity to confirm that the interval before the first fit was similar in the two cities (8/1). To make a direct comparison possible with missile injuries Professor Ritchie Russell kindly allowed me to abstract further details about fits in the first 8 weeks from the records of the series of gunshot wounds which had already been reported in respect of late traumatic epilepsy (Russell and Whitty, 1952); there were 73 with adequate information.

It is clear that the first week stands out as different, and as far and away the commonest week for epilepsy to begin (Fig. 3). This predominance can be expressed as the proportion of fits in the first 4 or 8

8/1   *Time of first fit within 8 weeks of injury*

Non-missile series	Week				
	1	2	3	4	5-8
Oxford (211)	165 78%	10 5%	4 2%	5 2%	27 13%
Glasgow (203)	175 86%	6 3%	4 2%	5 3%	13 6%
Total (414)	340 82%	16 4%	8 2%	10 2%	40 10%

weeks which began in the first week — 91% and 82% respectively for non-missile injuries (8/2). Alternatively the ratio can be calculated between the number of patients beginning epilepsy in the first week and the average number in each of the first 4 or 8 weeks — in each case this was 31 to 1; i.e. epilepsy after non-missile injury began in the first week 31 times more often than in any of the succeeding 7 weeks. In the missile series the first week again stood out but its predominance was not quite so marked, chiefly because of the number of fits beginning in the second week; this difference between the two types of injury was significant (8/3). The proportion in the first 4 and 8 weeks after missile injury which began in the first week was 77% and 64%; the ratio for first week to each of the next 7 weeks was 13 to 1.

Type of Fit (8/4)

Attacks limited to focal motor twitching, without the fit becoming generalised, were common only in the first week after injury; 41% of patients with epilepsy during this period had only such attacks. When epilepsy began in the next 7 weeks focal motor attacks occurred in only 17% of patients, and fits of this type were distinctly rare (3%) when epilepsy began after 3 months. Temporal lobe attacks were never encountered in the first week, although many of the patients were fully conscious when their epilepsy occurred and could well have reported the subjective elements of such attacks. In the next 7 weeks temporal lobe epilepsy occurred just as frequently as it did after 3 months.

8/2   *Time of first fit within 8 weeks of injury*

	Weeks 1-4	Week 1	Weeks 2-4		
			Total	Average per week	Ratio week 1 : 2/3/4
Non-missile	374	340 (91%)	34	11.0	31 : 1
Missile	61	47 (77%)	14	4.7	10 : 1

	Weeks 1-8	Week 1	Weeks 2-8		
			Total	Average per week	Ratio week 1 : 2/8
Non-missile	414	340 (82%)	74	11.0	31 : 1
Missile	73	47 (64%)	26	3.7	13 : 1

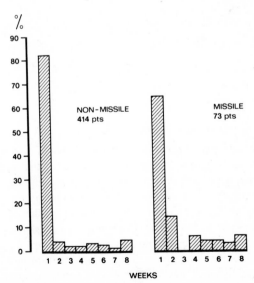

Fig. 3. Proportion of fits which began within 8 weeks of injury, by week of first fit.

8/3   *First week epilepsy after missile and non-missile injury*

	Total weeks 1-8	First week	
Non-missile (414)		340	82%
Missile (73)		47	64%
P			<0.001
	Total weeks 1 + 2	First week	
Non-missile (356)		340	96%
Missile (57)		47	82%
P			<0.001

8/4   *Type of fit at different intervals after injury*

	Focal motor attacks		Temporal lobe attacks	
Week 1	$^{140}/_{340}$	41%	$^{0}/_{340}$	0%
Weeks 2/8	$^{7}/_{41}$	17% }P < 0.01	$^{8}/_{41}$	20% }P < 0.001
> 3 months	$^{7}/_{218}$	3%	$^{48}/_{218}$	22%

Recurrence of Epilepsy in the Future

Patients with epilepsy beginning in weeks 2 to 8, and subsequently followed, proved to have a recurrence rate similar to that associated with epilepsy beginning more than 3 months after injury. Epilepsy in the first week had a significantly lower recurrence rate, both after non-missile and missile injuries (8/5). Recurrence is defined here as the development of any further epilepsy in the future. Reviewing the persistence of epilepsy 4 years after injury (i.e. continuing occurrence of seizures) Weiss and Caveness (1972) have shown a similar significant difference between patients whose epilepsy began in the first week compared with that developing later (8/6).

8/5   *Effect of time of first fit on recurrence*

Time of first fit	Recurrence rate			
	Non-missile		Missile	
Week 1	$^{59}/_{238}$	25% $\Big\}$ P < 0.001	$^{19}/_{41}$	46% $\Big\}$ P < 0.01
Weeks 2-8	$^{29}/_{41}$	71%	$^{19}/_{24}$	79%
After 3 months	$^{195}/_{254}$	77%	—	

8/6   *Epilepsy persisting at 4 years (mixed combat series)*
(Weiss and Caveness, 1972)

Time for first fit after injury	Persistence rate		
First week	$^{8}/_{26}$	31% $\Big\}$ P < 0.02	
1 week – 6 months	$^{19}/_{29}$	66% $\Big\}$ P NS	P < 0.01
> 6 months	$^{13}/_{18}$	72%	
All cases after first week	$^{32}/_{47}$	68%	

Different Influences on the Incidence of Early and Late Epilepsy

Interaction of various factors which influence the incidence of epilepsy at different periods after injury is complex and much of this volume is concerned with their analysis. From these analyses certain contrasts can be demonstrated between the factors which appear to be affecting the incidence of epilepsy during the first week and that occurring later, which would suggest that the mechanisms responsible for epilepsy in the first week may be different. The interpretation of these differences will be deferred until the chapters which deal fully with the factors influencing the incidence of early and late epilepsy, rather than anticipate by discussion out of context.

The increased liability of young children to develop early epilepsy is not reflected in late epilepsy, which young children are rather less liable to

8/7 *Different effects of certain factors on incidence of early and late epilepsy*

	Early		Late	
1. Age at injury				
< 5 years	$7/75$	9%	$24/149$	16%
> 5 years	$39/911$	4%	$161/832$	19%
P	< 0.05		NS	
2. Dural tearing				
(a) *Non-missile depressed fracture*				
Dura intact	$35/421$	8%	$20/303$	7%
Dura torn	$47/419$	11%	$73/309$	24%
P	NS		< 0.001	
(b) *Missile injuries* (Evans, 1963)				
Dura intact	$10/84$	12%	$12/84$	13%
Dura torn	$12/146$	8%	$58/146$	40%
P	NS		< 0.001	

develop (8/7). After non-missile depressed fractures (Jennett) and after missile injuries (Evans) early epilepsy occurs no more often when the dura is penetrated than when it is not; by contrast late epilepsy is significantly more common after dural penetration in both these types of injury (8/7). The effect of PTA shows some interesting contrasts between early and late epilepsy (8/8). The separate and combined influence of PTA and depressed fracture was different for early and for late epilepsy; either prolonged PTA or depressed fracture alone increased the incidence of early epilepsy, but the risk was no higher than when the two factors were combined. By contrast the incidence of late epilepsy was increased only when these two factors occurred together. After injuries without focal damage (no

8/8   *Effect of PTA and depressed fracture on early and late epilepsy*

	PTA < 24 hours		PTA > 24 hours		P
Early					
No depressed fracture	$^{16}/_{683}$	2%	$^{14}/_{137}$	10%	< 0.001
Depressed fracture	$^{65}/_{697}$	9%	$^{27}/_{230}$	12%	NS
P	< 0.001		NS		
Late					
No depressed fracture	$^{8}/_{125}$	6%	$^{9}/_{98}$	9%	NS
Depressed fracture	$^{45}/_{520}$	9%	$^{53}/_{166}$	32%	< 0.001
P	NS		< 0.001		
No depressed fracture or haematoma					
Early	$^{13}/_{665}$	2%	$^{10}/_{113}$	9%	< 0.001
Late	$^{5}/_{110}$	5%	$^{3}/_{79}$	4%	NS

depressed fracture or intracranial haematoma) a long PTA significantly increased the risk of early epilepsy but not that of late.

Conclusions

Evidence has been presented to support the view that epilepsy occurring within a week of injury is distinctly different from that occurring in the next few weeks. It confirms the view expressed by Earl Walker (1957); "it is generally considered that patients having attacks within a few weeks of the head injury usually have focal fits, and that the prognosis is better than when seizures develop later. The present study suggests, however, that such conclusions are justified only for first week epilepsy, and that the term "early epilepsy" should be used only for fits within the first week. As the present series has accumulated I have published a number of papers emphasising that early epilepsy should be so defined (Jennett and Lewin, 1960; Jennett, 1969a; Jennet, 1969b and Jennett, 1973). Apart

8/9 *Definitions of early epilepsy in reported series.*

Author	Year	Interval
Ascroft	1941	1 week
Whitty	1947	10 days
Russell and Whitty	1952	1 month
Phillips	1954	14 days
Caveness	1963	14 days
Evans	1963	18 days
Hendrick and Harris	1968	1 week
Courjon	1969	1 week
Stöwsand and Bues	1970	1 week
Adeloye and Odeku	1971	1 week
Rish and Caveness	1972	1 week
Weiss and Caveness	1972	1 week
Braakman	1972	1 week
Jamieson and Yelland	1972	1 week

from Weiss and Caveness (1972) no one appears to have produced evidence directed at supporting this definition, but in fact all recent publications on early traumatic epilepsy refer to fits in the first week after injury (8/9).

Chapter 9

INCIDENCE OF EARLY EPILEPSY

A direct estimate of the incidence can be made only in a series of consecutive hospital admissions such as the Oxford 1,000. In the event this yielded only 46 patients with early epilepsy so that many of the subgroups were too small for statistical analysis. It was for this reason that more patients with early epilepsy were sought (pages 16, 17). Having established that these additional patients closely resembled the Oxford series with early epilepsy (6/2), all the cases were treated for most purposes as one series. However, the Oxford series was used in some analyses for which it alone is valid, particularly to provide groups of patients without certain features, such as depressed fracture or haematoma, as explained previously (page 22). After the influence of various factors on the incidence of early epilepsy has been explored a calculation is made of the overall incidence of epilepsy, assuming the same frequency of occurrence of these factors as was found in the Oxford series.

Of the total series of patients with early epilepsy (9/1) 42% were under 16 years and a fifth were under 5 years of age when injured. About a quarter had depressed fracture, and another quarter an acute intracranial haematoma. Focal signs occurred in 25% and PTA of more than 24 hours in rather more than a third. A number were quite mildly injured, 26% having no focal signs, depressed fracture or haematoma, and with PTA not exceeding 24 hours.

Age at Injury

Early epilepsy was equally common in adults and in children as a whole (less than 16 years), but it occurred more frequently in young children (9/2). The age distribution for the series of early epilepsy showed significantly more patients under 5, and in the 5-15 age group, as compared with those injuries without epilepsy; this was also found by Stöwsand (1971) for children under 10 years (9/3); this is further evidence that young children are more liable to develop epilepsy. The first 3 years of life were disproportionately affected in the young children (Fig. 4).

After more severe injuries, as evidence by duration of PTA, fracture, haematoma or focal signs, early epilepsy was equally common in adults and children (9/4). But after less severe injuries epilepsy was more frequently found in children, and this proved to be mostly due to mild

9/1   *Features of injury in 417 pateints with early epilepsy*

< 5 years	78	19%
> 16 years	241	56%
PTA > 24 hours	$^{146}/_{366}$	40%
Focal signs	106	25%
Depressed fracture	98	25%
Intracranial haematoma	112	27%
No depressed fracture, haematoma or focal signs	176	42%

9/2   *Influence of age on incidence of early epilepsy*
(Oxford series)

< 5 years	$^{7}/_{75}$	9%
6-15 years	$^{4}/_{127}$	3%
16-25 years	$^{16}/_{279}$	6%
26-45 years	$^{10}/_{273}$	4%
46-65 years	$^{6}/_{151}$	4%
> 65 years	$^{3}/_{81}$	4%
< 16 years	$^{11}/_{202}$	5%
> 16 years	$^{35}/_{784}$	5%
P		NS
< 5 years	$^{7}/_{75}$	9%
> 5 years	$^{39}/_{911}$	4%
P		< 0.05

9/3   *Age distribution of injuries with and without early epilepsy*

	Without early epilepsy		With early epilepsy		P
1. *Present series*					
Total	950		417		<0.001
<5 years	68	7%	78	19%	<0.001
5-15 years	123	13%	98	24%	<0.001
>16 years	749	79%	241	58%	<0.001
2. *Stöwsand, 1971*					
Total	1000		107		<0.001
<10 years	188	19%	47	44%	<0.001
10-20 years	153	15%	16	15%	NS
>20 years	659	66%	44	41%	<0.001

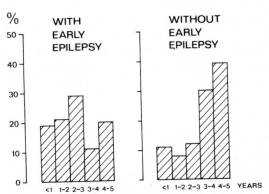

Fig. 4. Age at injury of young children, with and without early epilepsy.

injuries in young children. A mild injury might be defined as one not associated with unconsciousness or post-traumatic amnesia, but of injuries so defined in the Oxford series one in five had suffered either a depressed fracture or had developed an intracranial haematoma. An injury was therefore defined as *trivial* only if it had caused no initial unconsciousness or PTA and it was complicated by neither depressed fracture nor acute intracranial haematoma. The proportion of such trivial injuries was approximately similar in those with and without early epilepsy, and the

9/4   *Incidence of early epilepsy in children and adults with various features*

Features	< 16 years		> 16 years		P
PTA > 24 hours	$2/20$	10%	$16/134$	12%	NS
Linear fracture	$3/78$	4%	$14/194$	7%	NS
Depressed fracture	$49/459$	11%	$47/488$	10%	NS
Haematoma	$17/68$	25%	$95/352$	27%	NS
Neurological signs	$8/49$	16%	$2/228$	10%	NS
PTA < 24 hours	$9/173$	5%	$11/556$	2%	< 0.05
No fracture	$6/92$	7%	$7/455$	2%	< 0.01
No depressed fracture	$9/170$	5%	$28/735$	4%	NS
No haematoma	$8/193$	4%	$25/735$	3%	NS
No neurological signs	$3/189$	2%	$4/430$	1%	NS

9/5   *Frequency of trivial injuries–patients with and without early epilepsy*

Age	With no early epilepsy		With early epilepsy		P
< 5 years	$20/68$	29%	$17/78$	22%	NS
5-15 years	$16/123$	13%	$8/98$	8%	NS
> 16 years	$43/760$	6%	$7/241$	3%	NS

9/6   *Frequency of trivial injuries at different ages*

< 5 years	$37/144$	26%	$P < 0.001$
> 5 years	$74/1259$	6%	$P < 0.001$
5-15 years	$24/220$	11%	$P < 0.001$
< 16 years	$61/364$	17%	$P < 0.001$
> 16 years	$50/1039$	5%	

9/7 *Incidence of early epilepsy after trivial injuries (Oxford series)*

< 5 years	$^4/_{24}$	17%	
6-15 years	$^0/_{16}$		
16-25 years	$^1/_{13}$	$^1/_{59}$	2%
> 25 years	$^0/_{30}$		
P		< 0.001	

age distribution was also similar (9/5). Such injuries were significantly more common under the age of 5 years, accounting for a quarter of young children admitted (9/6). In older children trivial injuries were significantly less common than in young children, but still occurred more frequently than in adults. Two studies of patients with early epilepsy likewise found mild injuries more common in children. Stöwsand (1971) found that 31% of children (under 13 years) were mildly injured compared with 7% of adults (P < 0.02). Hendrick and Harris (1968) reported children with early epilepsy and 75% had trivial or mild injuries.

The incidence of early epilepsy after trivial injuries was higher in young children; in the Oxford series of 83 trivial injuries 17% of the under 5's developed early epilepsy compared with 2% over the age of 5 (9/7). This suggests that after a trivial injury over the age of 5 epilepsy might be a rare occurrence but in the enlarged series of 32 patients with early epilepsy after trivial injury 15 (47%) were over 5 years old. However, all 7 adults with early epilepsy had "immediate" fits, an unusual type of traumatic epilepsy (see page 67). It remains true therefore that early epilepsy which was not immediate after trivial injury was confined to children (under 16 years).

Severity of Injury

The various features considered to indicate a more severe injury probably reflect different kinds of brain damage. After non-missile injuries it is frequently difficult to deduce from clinical features either the site or the degree of damage which has been sustained. The evidence for regarding the duration of PTA as a reflection of the degree of diffuse brain damage has already been presented (pages 6-7). It seems possible that linear skull fracture may also be indicative of some degree of diffuse brain damage; certainly patients without either PTA or linear fracture might be regarded as having sustained a lesser degree of diffuse brain damage than those with other types of injury. On the other hand depressed fractures, acute intracranial haematoma and focal (hemisphere) neurological signs are each indicative of local brain damage. Whilst it is impossible to conclude that patients without these features do not have any local brain damage it is of interest to compare the incidence of epilepsy in those with and without these signs.

Injuries which were more severe or complicated, as evidenced by each of these factors, were associated with an increased risk of epilepsy (9/8).

9/8 *Incidence of early epilepsy after injuries with various features*

Feature	Feature present		Feature absent		P
PTA > 24 hours	$18/154$	12%	$20/729$	3%	< 0.001
Linear fracture	$17/272$	6%	$13/547$	2%	< 0.01
Depressed fracture	$96/947$	10%	$13/547$	2%	< 0.001
Intracranial haematoma	$112/420$	27%	$33/928$	4%	< 0.001
Focal signs	$23/182$	13%	$15/714$	2%	< 0.001

9/9 *Incidence of early epilepsy with various features*

Feature	Feature present		Feature absent		P
< 16 years					
PTA > 24 hours	$2/20$	10%	$9/173$	5%	NA
Linear fracture	$3/78$	4%	$6/92$	7%	NS
Depressed fracture	$49/459$	11%	$9/170$	5%	< 0.05
Intracranial haematoma	$17/68$	25%	$8/193$	4%	< 0.001
Neurological signs	$8/49$	16%	$3/189$	2%	< 0.001
> 16 years					
PTA > 24 hours	$16/134$	12%	$11/556$	2%	< 0.001
Linear fracture	$14/194$	7%	$7/455$	2%	< 0.001
Depressed fracture	$47/488$	10%	$28/735$	4%	< 0.001
Intracranial haematoma	$95/352$	27%	$25/735$	3%	< 0.001
Neurological signs	$2/228$	10%	$4/430$	1%	< 0.001

In adults this increased risk was more consistent than in children (9/9), which confirms that children are prone to early epilepsy after mild injuries.

Post-traumatic Amnesia

The association between early epilepsy and injuries associated with more than 24 hours PTA (9/8) was confirmed by the increased frequency of prolonged PTA in the early epilepsy series, as compared with the Oxford injuries without epilepsy (9/10). The relationship between epilepsy and PTA can be explored in more detail in the Oxford series. No difference was found in the incidence of early epilepsy after injuries associated with PTA lasting 1-7 days as compared with more than 7 days; nor between those with PTA lasting less than 1 hour as compared with 1-24 hours. But after the less severe injuries epilepsy was significantly *more* frequent when there was *no* PTA than when amnesia was definite but lasted less than 24 hours (9/11). Some confirmation of this association is found in the different distribution of PTA in injuries with and without early epilepsy. As would be expected patients with prolonged PTA (1-7 days and more than 7 days) were more frequent in the epilepsy series whilst the opposite

9/10   *Frequency of injuries with >24 hours PTA*

No early epilepsy	$136/845$	16%
With early epilepsy	$159/384$	41%
P		< 0.001

9/11   *Influence of PTA on incidence of early epilepsy*
(Oxford Series)

PTA					
NIL	$7/108$	6%			
< 1 hour	$7/414$	2%	$13/621$	2%	P < 0.01
1-24 hours	$6/207$	3%			
1-7 days	$7/64$	11%			
> 7 days	$11/90$	12%			

was the case for amnesia which was definite but less than 24 hours; patients with no PTA were equally represented in these two groups (9/12). Among patients with less than 24 hours PTA those with no amnesia were significantly more common in the epilepsy series (9/13). In their study of children with epilepsy Hendrick and Harris made a similar observation, in that it was commoner to find no loss of consciousness than brief loss of consciousness in those developing epilepsy. They explained this by referring to Walker's contention that brief periods of unconsciousness were probably related to brain stem injury, which would not be likely to occasion epilepsy. An alternative explanation, for some of the cases, may be the occurrence of depressed fracture or intracranial haematoma in patients without amnesia. A substantial minority of patients with no amnesia were complicated by depressed fracture or haematoma, both in those with early epilepsy (37% complicated), and in those without (23% complicated); corresponding proportions of those with amnesia, but less than 24 hours PTA in duration, were 28% with early epilepsy and 6% of those without (9/14).

The effect of PTA on the incidence of early epilepsy is summarised in

9/12   *Frequency distribution of PTA in series with and without early epilepsy*

PTA	Without early epilepsy 843		With early epilepsy 352		P
Nil	101	12%	51	15%	NS
Up to 24 hours	606	72%	173	49%	<0.001
1-7 days	57	7%	49	14%	<0.001
>7 days	79	9%	79	22%	<0.001

9/13   *Frequency of "no amnesia" in injuries with up to 24 hours PTA*

Injuries without early epilepsy	$^{101}/_{707}$	14%
Early epilepsy series	$^{51}/_{224}$	23%
P	<0.01	

9/15 which shows that although prolonged amnesia consistently increased the early epilepsy rate it did not do so in injuries already associated with a high risk (children, or patients with depressed fracture, haematoma or focal signs). It was of most significance in adults and patients with neither depressed fracture nor haematoma, when epilepsy was unusual unless PTA exceeded 24 hours. These findings are at variance with those of Evans (1963); reporting combat injuries from Korea he found PTA to bear no relation to the incidence of early epilepsy after non-missile injuries, but to be significant after missile injuries.

Linear Fracture

Early epilepsy is significantly commoner after injuries associated with linear fracture than in those with no fracture (9/16). This is reflected in the higher incidence of linear fracture in the early epilepsy series compared with other injuries (9/17). The site of the linear fracture proved not to

9/14 *Frequency of depressed fracture or haematoma in injuries with PTA < 24 hours*

	Without early epilepsy		With early epilepsy	
No PTA	$^{23}/_{101}$	23%	$^{19}/_{51}$	37%
PTA up to 24 hours	$^{34}/_{606}$	6%	$^{48}/_{173}$	28%

9/15 *Influence of PTA on incidence of early epilepsy*

	PTA < 24 hours		PTA > 24 hours		P
< 16 years	$^9/_{173}$	5%	$^2/_{20}$	10%	NS
> 16 years	$^{11}/_{556}$	2%	$^{16}/_{34}$	12%	< 0.001
Depressed fracture	$^{65}/_{697}$	9%	$^{27}/_{230}$	14%	NS
Haematoma	$^{36}/_{136}$	26%	$^{62}/_{210}$	30%	NS
Focal signs	$^{14}/_{160}$	9%	$^{16}/_{117}$	14%	NS
No depressed fracture or haematoma	$^{13}/_{665}$	2%	$^{10}/_{113}$	9%	< 0.001

affect the incidence of early epilepsy significantly although epilepsy was less common after linear occipital fracture (9/18).

Depressed Fracture

This significantly increased the incidence of early epilepsy both in children and adults (9/19). When the epilepsy rate was already high, because of prolonged PTA or focal signs, depressed fracture did not add further to the risk. The site of fracture did not influence the incidence of early epilepsy significantly; further details about this and other interactions are discussed in Chapter 16.

9/16   *Effect of skull fracture on incidence of early epilepsy*

No fracture	$13/581$	2%
Linear fracture	$24/331$	7%
P	<0.001	

9/17   *Frequency of linear fractures with and without early epilepsy*

Injuries with no early epilepsy	$255/858$	30%
With early epilepsy	$149/386$	39%
P	<0.01	

9/18   *Effect of site of linear fracture on early epilepsy*

Temporo-parietal	$16/173$	9%
Frontal	$6/95$	6%
P	NS	
Occipital	$2/63$	2%
Other sites	$22/268$	8%
P	NS	

Acute Intracranial Haematoma

This significantly increased the risk of early epilepsy, more so with intradural than extradural haematoma. This applied to both adults and children and whether PTA was prolonged or not (9/20). Further details are discussed in Chapter 17.

Neurological Signs

In the original Oxford series some neurological sign was recorded in 30% of the surviving injuries; in two thirds of cases with signs these included those associated with damage to the cerebral hemisphere (motor or

9/19 *Effect of depressed fracture on incidence of early epilepsy*

	No depressed fracture		Depressed fracture		P
All cases	$37/912$	4%	$96/947$	10%	<0.001
<16 years	$9/170$	5%	$49/459$	11%	<0.05
>16 years	$28/735$	4%	$47/488$	10%	<0.001
<24 hours PTA	$16/683$	2%	$65/697$	9%	<0.001
>24 hours PTA	$14/137$	10%	$27/230$	12%	NS
No focal signs	$8/663$	1%	$71/756$	9%	<0.001
With focal signs	$22/169$	13%	$25/192$	13%	NS

9/20 *Effect of haematoma on incidence of early epilepsy*

	No haematoma		Haematoma		P
All cases	$33/928$	4%	$112/420$	27%	<0.001
<16 years	$8/193$	4%	$17/68$	25%	<0.001
>16 years	$25/735$	3%	$95/352$	27%	<0.001
<24 hours PTA	$17/711$	2%	$36/136$	26%	<0.001
>24 hours PTA	$14/130$	11%	$62/210$	30%	<0.001

sensory hemiparesis, hemianopia or dysphasia). Such focal signs were not significantly more common in the series with early epilepsy, or with depressed fracture than in the Oxford injuries as a whole, but were more common in association with acute haematoma (9/21). Patients with focal signs more often developed early epilepsy than did those with other signs (9/22). However, focal signs did not increase the incidence of early epilepsy after depressed fracture or after acute haematoma, both of which are already associated with a high risk of early epilepsy (9/23). Information about the interaction of age and of PTA on the incidence of early epilepsy in patients with and without signs is available only for the

9/21   *Frequency of focal signs in different series*

Oxford series	$182/896$	20%
Early epilepsy	$97/392$	25%
Depressed fractures	$192/948$	20%
Haematomas	$175/420$	42%

9/22   *Incidence of early epilepsy after focal and other signs*

Focal (hemisphere) signs	$23/182$	13%
Other signs	$7/95$	7%
P	NS	

9/23   *Effect of hemisphere (focal) signs on incidence of early epilepsy*

	No focal signs		Focal signs		P
All cases (Oxford series)	$15/714$	2%	$23/182$	13%	<0.001
Depressed fracture	$71/756$	9%	$12/192$	13%	NS
Haematoma	$62/245$	25%	$50/75$	29%	NS

group with any signs; analysis indicates that signs significantly increase the risk of epilepsy in both adults and children, and whether or not PTA is prolonged (9/24). As two thirds of patients with any signs have in fact focal signs it is probable that the same relationships would apply to patients with focal signs.

Subarachnoid Haemorrhage

It was not the practice in Oxford to perform routine lumbar puncture after head injury. Indeed only 174 (19%) of survivors were punctured. Seventy-one per cent of these had blood-stained fluid and it was clear that the patients punctured were those suspected of having blood, and they might thereby be suspected also of including a high proportion of more severe injuries; however, 41% had no fracture, and 47% had less than 24 hours PTA. The number of punctures with negative findings was too small for comparison, and those with proved SAH are therefore compared with the rest of the series — for which it was assumed only that subarachnoid haemorrhage was "not proven" (to borrow a usefully ambiguous phrase from Scots law). In the event subarachnoid haemorrhage was associated with an increased incidence of early epilepsy, particularly after injuries associated without fracture or with less than 24 hours PTA (9/25).

Family History of Epilepsy

Information about whether or not first degree relatives suffered from epilepsy was available in only 396 patients. A family history was somewhat more common in those with early epilepsy, and this was more obvious in adults (9/26).

9/24   *Effect of neurological signs (any) on incidence of early epilepsy*

	No signs		Any signs		P
All cases	$8/619$	1%	$30/277$	11%	<0.001
<16 years	$3/189$	2%	$8/49$	16%	<0.001
>16 years	$5/430$	1%	$22/228$	10%	<0.001
<24 hours PTA	$6/583$	1%	$14/160$	9%	<0.001
>24 hours PTA	$2/55$	4%	$16/117$	14%	<0.05

9/25 *Effect of subarachnoid haemorrhage (SAH) on incidence of early epilepsy*

	SAH absent or not proven		With SAH		P
All cases	$^{26}/_{759}$	3%	$^{12}/_{124}$	10%	<0.01
<16 years	$^{8}/_{181}$	4%	$^{3}/_{12}$	25%	<0.01
>16 years	$^{18}/_{580}$	3%	$^{9}/_{110}$	8%	<0.02
>24 hours PTA	$^{14}/_{672}$	2%	$^{6}/_{57}$	11%	<0.001
<24 hours PTA	$^{12}/_{89}$	14%	$^{6}/_{65}$	9%	NS
No fracture	$^{8}/_{497}$	2%	$^{5}/_{50}$	10%	<0.001
With fracture	$^{18}/_{264}$	7%	$^{7}/_{72}$	10%	NS

9/26 *Frequency of positive family history*

	No early epilepsy		With early epilepsy		P
All cases	$^{13}/_{264}$	5%	$^{10}/_{132}$	8%	NS
<16 years	$^{10}/_{100}$	10%	$^{5}/_{76}$	7%	NS
>16 years	$^{3}/_{164}$	2%	$^{5}/_{56}$	9%	NS

Overall Incidence

The original series of 1,000 in Oxford yielded 46 cases of first week epilepsy. That was a prospective study of patients admitted to a hospital where the neurosurgeon was immediately involved in their care and it was therefore unlikely that early epilepsy would be overlooked. It was suspected that this might result in a higher than usual incidence being recorded. Since then many more cases of depressed fracture and intracranial haematoma from other cities have been collected; in the event the epilepsy rate in these additional cases is similar to that observed in the Oxford series, indicating that there was no bias in that series. Moreover the additional cases with early epilepsy have been shown to correspond closely with those in the original series (6/2). There is therefore no reason to amend the original estimate of about 5% for early epilepsy in head injuries admitted to hospital. Courjon has subsequently reported first week epilepsy in 4% of 1,000 injuries. Because the incidence is higher in children it might be expected that a children's hospital would produce a higher rate, and indeed Stöwsand and Bues (1970) have reported early epilepsy in 7% of 814 children under 15 years of age, compared with 2% in 2,354 adults. However, Hendrick and Harris (1968) found only 5% with epilepsy in 4,195 head injured children under the age of 15; but the rate was 7% in children under 5, and 11% for injuries in the first year of life (excluding birth injuries). Early epilepsy is also likely to be discovered more frequently in neurosurgical units which selectively admit patients with more severe and complicated injuries, which have been shown to be associated with a higher than average incidence of early epilepsy.

Although only a small proportion of injuries are complicated by epilepsy the prevalence of head injury makes early traumatic epilepsy quite a common event. On the basis of a hospital admission rate of 100,000 head injuries per annum, it is probable that some 5,000 patients develop early epilepsy in hospital each year in Britain. For missile injuries the early epilepsy rate is not dissimilar and seems not to have changed through successive wars.

Chapter 10

CHARACTER OF EARLY EPILEPSY

Three characteristics of early epilepsy are considered — the type of fit (focal or not), the interval after injury until the first fit, and the number of fits occurring during the first week. The association between these aspects of early epilepsy and various features of injury is first explored and then the interaction between these characteristics.

Types of Fit

Some focal feature was recognised in at least one of the early fits suffered by 57% of 411 patients with early epilepsy (10/1). In 75% of patients with focal epilepsy only focal motor attacks were suffered, these accounting for 43% of all patients with early epilepsy. Age did not affect these proportions. Stöwsand's findings were similar in his 102 patients with early epilepsy, 64% having focal attacks, of which 79% were focal motor. Evans (1963) reported 63% of focal attacks in non-missile injuries and 79% for missile; Rish and Caveness (1972) likewise found a higher proportion of focal attacks (68%) after missile injuries.

Focal attacks occurred somewhat more often when PTA exceeded 24 hours (10/2). Only in adults were focal attacks significantly more common with prolonged PTA (10/3).

10/1   *Effect of age on type of fit*

Age	All focal	Focal motor only
All ages	233	175
	57%	43%
< 5 years (79)	46	34
	58%	43%
5-15 years (102)	58	48
	57%	47%
> 16 years (230)	129	93
	56%	40%

10/2   *Effect of PTA on type of fit*

PTA	Focal		Focal motor	
Nil (55)	30	55%	22	40%
<1 hour (105)	52	50%	36	34%
1-24 hours (67)	32	48%	23	32%
1-7 days (52)	29	56%	18	35%
>7 days (86)	59	69%	49	57%

Focal: $114/227$ 50% ; $88/138$ 64% ; $P < 0.05$

Focal motor: $81/227$ 36% ; $67/133$ 50% ; $P < 0.01$

10/3   *Effect of PTA on proportion of focal attacks*

Age	PTA <24 hours		PTA >24 hours		P
All ages	$^{118}/_{233}$	51%	$^{99}/_{152}$	65%	<0.01
<5 years	$^{32}/_{57}$	56%	$^{6}/_{10}$	60%	NS
5-15 years	$^{36}/_{69}$	52%	$^{20}/_{30}$	67%	NS
>16 years	$^{50}/_{107}$	47%	$^{73}/_{112}$	65%	<0.01

10/4   *Type of early epilepsy with different features of injury*

	% with focal attacks	
No depressed fracture	$^{164}/_{286}$	57%
Depressed fracture	$^{56}/_{100}$	56%
P	NS	
No haematoma	$^{173}/_{324}$	53%
Haematoma	$^{70}/_{112}$	63%
P	NS	
	% with focal motor	
No depressed fracture	$^{46}/_{100}$	46%
Depressed fracture	$^{121}/_{286}$	42%
P	NS	
No haematoma	$^{127}/_{324}$	39%
Haematoma	$^{58}/_{112}$	52%
P	NS	

10/5 *Effect of age on time of first fit after injury*

Age	Onset first hour		Onset 1-24 hours		Onset > 24 hours	
All ages (407)	115	28%	136	33%	156	38%
<16 years (179)	65	36% } $P<0.001$	74	41% } $P<0.01$	40	22% } $P<0.001$
>16 years (228)	50	22%	62	27%	116	51%
<5 years (78)	24	31% } P NS	36	46% } P NS	18	23% } P NS
5-15 years (101)	41	40%	38	38%	22	22%

Focal epilepsy was no more common after depressed fracture, which contrasts with Stöwsand's report that 14 of his 15 patients with early epilepsy after depressed fracture had focal attacks. After acute intracranial haematoma focal epilepsy was somewhat more common, as were focal motor attacks (10/4).

Time of Onset (Interval from Injury to First Fit)

The first early fit occurred within 24 hours of injury in 61% of patients; in rather less than half of these it had happened within the first hour. In children epilepsy more often began during the first day, and also more often within the first hour after injury; there was no significant difference between younger and older children (10/5). These findings are somewhat at variance with Stöwsand's in whose general series 74% began in the first day; and with Hendrick and Harris' childhood series, of which 69% began within 24 hours.

When PTA was less than 24 hours epilepsy more often began in the first hour and less often after the first day; PTA did not influence the proportion of early epilepsy beginning in the 1-24 hour period (10/6).

10/6   *Effect of PTA on interval to first early fit*

PTA	First hour		1-24 hours		>24 hours	
<24 hours (232)	83	36%	79	34%	70	30%
>24 hours (150)	25	17%	47	31%	78	52%
P	<0.001		NS		<0.001	

10/7   *Effect of PTA on proportion with onset on first day*

Age	PTA <24 hours		PTA >24 hours		P
All ages	$162/232$	70%	$72/150$	48%	<0.001
<5 years	$48/57$	84%	$4/10$	40%	<0.001
5-15 years	$55/69$	80%	$21/30$	70%	NS
>16 years	$59/107$	55%	$47/112$	42%	NS

10/8 *Effect of PTA on proportion of fits in first day*

Nil	$43/55$	78%			
< 1 hour	$73/104$	70%	$159/226$ 70%		
1-24 hours	$43/67$	64%			$P < 0.001$
1-7 days	$27/52$	52%	$67/136$ 49%		
> 7 days	$40/84$	48%			

10/9 *Time of onset of early epilepsy with different features of injury*

	% onset < 1 hour	
No depressed fracture	$69/282$	25%
Depressed fracture	$39/100$	39%
P	< 0.01	

No haematoma	$107/321$	33%
Haematoma	$11/108$	10%
P	< 0.001	

	% onset > 24 hours	
No depressed fracture	$118/282$	42%
Depressed fracture	$28/100$	28%
P	< 0.01	

No haematoma	$95/321$	30%
Haematoma	$74/110$	69%
P	< 0.001	

10/10   *Effect of age on number of early fits*

	Single		Status	
All ages (405)	143	35%	46	11%
< 5 years (77)	18	23% ⎫	17	22% ⎫
>5 years (328)	125	38% ⎬ <0.02	29	9% ⎬ <0.001
5-15 years (100)	43	43% ⎫	12	12% ⎫
>16 years (228)	82	36% ⎬ NS	17	8% ⎬ NS

More detailed analysis revealed little difference within the two PTA groups (10/7). Although this relationship was observed in all age groups it was significant only for the under fives (10/8). Early fits after depressed fracture more often began in the first hour and less often after 24 hours, whilst after intracranial haematoma the opposite was observed (10/9). This latter relationship has also been reported by Stöwsand (with haematoma 31% of fits in the first day, without 83%).

Number of Fits

Only one fit occurred during the first week in 35% of patients but 11% had status epilepticus; this corresponds to Stöwsand's report in which 42% had single fits and 23% status. In children under 5 years single fits were less common, whilst status occurred in 22% compared with 8% of adults (10/10). This is at variance with Hendrick and Harris' observation that "almost all" their children had only a single fit. When PTA was less than 24 hours a single fit was more common, but this difference was significant only in adults (10/11). Stöwsand likewise found single fits more often after milder injuries than severe (27%). After trivial injuries early fits were only slightly more often single (42%) than after other injuries (35%), although Stöwsand reported that 87% of fits after trivial injuries were

10/11   *Effect of PTA on proportion of single fits*

	PTA < 24 hours		PTA > 24 hours		P
All ages	$^{99}/_{231}$	43%	$^{38}/_{149}$	26%	< 0.001
< 5 years	$^{16}/_{57}$	28%	$^{0}/_{10}$	0%	NS
5-15 years	$^{33}/_{69}$	48%	$^{9}/_{30}$	30%	NS
> 16 years	$^{50}/_{107}$	47%	$^{29}/_{112}$	26%	< 0.001

10/12   *Number of attacks after depressed fracture or acute haematoma*

	% with single attack	
No depressed fracture	$^{82}/_{280}$	29%
Depressed fracture	$^{52}/_{99}$	53%
P	< 0.001	
No haematoma	$^{124}/_{320}$	39%
Haematoma	$^{24}/_{110}$	22%
P	< 0.01	

	% with status	
No depressed fracture	$^{33}/_{280}$	12%
Depressed fracture	$^{7}/_{99}$	7%
P	NS	
No haematoma	$^{35}/_{320}$	11%
Haematoma	$^{14}/_{110}$	13%
P	NS	

single. Duration of PTA did not appear to affect the incidence of status which was likewise unaffected by depressed fracture or intracranial haematoma. These last two complications had opposite effects on the incidence of single fits, which were more common after depressed fracture and less common after haematoma (10/12).

Interaction between Characteristics

Single attacks were more likely to be non-focal, as were fits which began in the first hour or after the first day. Those with status were more likely to be focal (10/13).

10/13 *Type of fit in different kinds of early epilepsy*

Feature	% with focal attacks		P
	Feature present	Feature absent	
Single attack	$^{57}/_{143}$ 40%	$^{171}/_{262}$ 65%	<0.001
Status	$^{37}/_{45}$ 80%	$^{191}/_{357}$ 54%	<0.001
Onset: first hour	$^{48}/_{115}$ 42%	$^{182}/_{292}$ 62%	<0.001
Onset: >24 hours	$^{108}/_{251}$ 43%	$^{122}/_{156}$ 78%	<0.001

10/14 *Time of first fit in different kinds of early epilepsy*

Feature	% with onset in first hour after injury		P
	Feature present	Feature absent	
Single fit	$^{65}/_{141}$ 46%	$^{49}/_{261}$ 19%	<0.001
Status	$^{12}/_{46}$ 26%	$^{102}/_{356}$ 29%	NS
Focal fit	$^{48}/_{230}$ 21%	$^{67}/_{177}$ 38%	<0.001
	% with onset >24 hours after injury		
Single fit	$^{28}/_{141}$ 20%	$^{126}/_{261}$ 48%	<0.001
Status	$^{24}/_{46}$ 52%	$^{130}/_{356}$ 36%	NS
Focal fit	$^{122}/_{230}$ 53%	$^{34}/_{177}$ 19%	<0.001

10/15 *Number of attacks in different kinds of early epilepsy*

Feature	% with single fits		P
	Feature present	Feature absent	
Focal fits	$^{57}/_{228}$ 25%	$^{86}/_{177}$ 49%	<0.001
Onset: first hour	$^{65}/_{114}$ 57%	$^{72}/_{288}$ 26%	<0.001
Onset: > 24 hours	$^{28}/_{154}$ 18%	$^{113}/_{248}$ 46%	<0.001
	% with status		
Focal fits	$^{37}/_{228}$ 16%	$^{9}/_{177}$ 5%	<0.001
Onset: first hour	$^{12}/_{114}$ 11%	$^{33}/_{288}$ 12%	NS
Onset: >24 hours	$^{24}/_{154}$ 16%	$^{21}/_{248}$ 9%	NS

Single attacks were more likely to occur in the first hour (46%) and were less often delayed beyond 24 hours (20%). The opposite held for status — 26% in the first hour and 52% after 24 hours (10/14). Focal attacks were more often delayed beyond the first day (53%), and only 21% began in the first hour. More than half the patients with status developed epilepsy after the first day and only 27% in the first hour.

Half the patients with non-focal attacks had only a single attack, compared with a quarter of those with focal epilepsy; more than half of those with a fit in the first hour had a single attack only, compared with less than a fifth of those beginning after 24 hours. Status was more common with focal attacks, and when epilepsy began more than 24 hours after injury (10/15).

Chapter 11

SIGNIFICANCE OF EARLY EPILEPSY

Those authors who have recommended that fits soon after injury should be excluded from discussions about traumatic epilepsy appear usually to have done so because seizures in this period were believed to be of little importance. It is best to consider separately the significance of such seizures for the *immediate* management of the patient in the early post-traumatic period soon after epilepsy has occurred, and their significance for the *future*.

Immediate Significance

As Evidence of an Intracranial Complication

Both intracranial haematoma and infection are not uncommonly associated with fits. The question is whether the development of epilepsy is in itself important evidence in favour of such a complication and whether it justifies further action, such as transfer to another centre, the initiation of investigations, or even the performance of burr holes. These complications are in fact much more consistently associated with other features, such as deterioration of conscious level; however, a fit is so much more dramatic an event that not infrequently it is what draws attention to the possibility of a complication.

In the unselected Oxford series 28% of patients with early epilepsy had an intracranial haematoma. Two thirds of these were patients with acute subdural intracranial haematoma, 49% of whom developed early epilepsy. However, these patients were already seriously ill with focal signs and altered consciousness and the occurrence of epilepsy was an incidental event of little diagnostic significance. It is of more concern to discover how often epilepsy heralds an extradural haematoma, which frequently develops after a lucid interval or even when there has been no initial loss of consciousness. In fact only 10% of patients with extradural haematoma had early epilepsy and in a third of these the first fit did not occur until after the evacuation of the clot. In the present series of patients with early epilepsy less than 2% proved to be developing an extradural haematoma at the time of their first fit, and even in these there were always other signs pointing to a complication. Among patients who develop early epilepsy after injuries associated with no amnesia only a small proportion (8%) had haematoma. It seems reasonable therefore to conclude that the occurrence of a fit is in itself no reason for strongly suspecting an intracranial haematoma. Unless there are other features pointing to this or any other intracranial complication epilepsy does not justify further investigation and certainly not exploration.

Dangers of Status

Although status occurred in only 11% of all patients with early epilepsy, 22% of children under the age of 5 were affected. Status carries considerable potential hazards, and active treatment must be promptly instituted. At least one childhood death from status epilepticus following a mild head injury has been reported (Small and Woolff, 1957). However, all five children with status after mild injuries in a recent report made a good recovery (Grand, 1974). Mortality was no higher in those with status than in other types of early epilepsy in the present series.

The possibility of persisting brain damage in survivors after status should be remembered in assessing the possible significance of traumatic epilepsy. No data is available about this for the present series.

Mortality

Patients with early epilepsy had a higher mortality (9%) than those who did not (5%), and epilepsy was commoner in fatal injuries (9%) than in non-fatal (4%). This apparent relationship between mortality and epilepsy was due almost wholly to the association between acute intracranial haematoma and both early epilepsy and increased mortality. Almost two thirds of deaths after early epilepsy were associated with intracranial haematoma, which occurred in only 16% of fatal head injuries without early epilepsy.

Significance for the Future

In 1932 Riddoch wrote that "convulsions in the state of concussion" were no indication of the likelihood of late epilepsy, and in 1954 Jasper likewise wrote that "convulsions in the acute stage of the reaction to trauma" had little significance in regard to late epilepsy. Authors who exclude fits occurring in the early days or weeks after injury from their assessment of traumatic epilepsy imply that they regard seizures at this stage as of no lasting consequence. However, both Wagstaff (1928) and Symonds (1935) held that although early fits might not often recur they did indicate an increased risk of epilepsy in the future, and Whitty (1947) came to a similar conclusion about missile injuries.

Analysis of the original Oxford series (Jennett and Lewin, 1960; Jennett, 1962) indicated that late epilepsy was significantly more common in patients who had suffered early epilepsy. That statement was based on the follow-up of only 35 patients who suffered early epilepsy; it is now possible to report that the follow-up of a further 200 patients has sustained the original finding. Since 1962 there have been a number of published reports which confirm the significance of early epilepsy in relation to late epilepsy (11/1).

The patients followed after early epilepsy were shown to correspond closely to the survivors from the original series with early epilepsy, which indicated that there had not been a bias towards more complicated or severe injuries among those successfully followed (6/5). Late epilepsy occurred significantly more often in those patients who had suffered early epilepsy than in those who had not; this late epilepsy rate was somewhat lower in children than in adults (11/2). These findings correspond closely

11/1   *Incidence of LATE epilepsy after early epilepsy*

	After early epilepsy		No early epilepsy	
All ages				
Jennett	$^{59}/_{238}$	25%	$^{29}/_{868}$	3%
Courjon	—	13%	—	
Stöwsand	$^{14}/_{71}$	20%	$^{6}/_{468}$	1%
Adults				
Jennett	$^{39}/_{120}$	33%	$^{22}/_{663}$	3%
Stöwsand	$^{7}/_{31}$	23%	—	
Evans	$^{5}/_{14}$	36%	$^{7}/_{134}$	5%
Weiss and Caveness	$^{8}/_{26}$	31%	—	
Children				
Jennett	$^{20}/_{118}$	17%	$^{8}/_{230}$	4%
Stöwsand	$^{8}/_{40}$	20%	$^{8}/_{230}$	4%
Hendrick and Harris	$^{37}/_{174}$	21%	—	2%

with other recently reported series, which likewise indicate a somewhat lower recurrence rate in children (11/1). It must be emphasised that the incidence of late epilepsy in children is still highly significant by comparison with children who do not have early epilepsy, and this runs counter to general paediatric opinion, as far as this can be deduced from text-books and current practice. There appears to be among paediatricians a tendency to regard a fit in the first week after injury as not dissimilar from other types of symptomatic epilepsy associated with acutely developing and rapidly resolving clinical conditions. In this regard the place of febrile convulsions is a special one and has attracted a good deal of investigation. A parallel might reasonably be sought between early traumatic epilepsy and febrile convulsions, although traumatic epilepsy does not show the relation to family history nor the particular age distribution of febrile convulsions. However, it is interesting that the weight of opinion appears now to accept that children who have febrile convulsions do have an increased risk of epilepsy in the future, as has now been shown after traumatic epilepsy.

11/2   Incidence of LATE epilepsy

(a) Influence of early epilepsy

	All cases		< 16 years		> 16 years	
No early epilepsy	$^{29}/_{868}$	3%	$^{8}/_{230}$	4%	$^{21}/_{638}$	3%
After early epilepsy	$^{59}/_{238}$	25%	$^{20}/_{118}$	17%	$^{39}/_{120}$	33%
P	< 0.001		< 0.001		< 0.001	

(b) After early epilepsy at different ages

< 5 years	$^{8}/_{42}$	19%	< 16 years	$^{20}/_{118}$	17%
> 5 years	$^{51}/_{196}$	26%	> 16 years	$^{39}/_{120}$	33%
P	NS		P	< 0.01	
	5-15 years	$^{12}/_{76}$	16%		

The influence of early epilepsy on the incidence of late epilepsy is seen in several different types of injury (11/3). Its effect is most striking after injuries which are uncomplicated by either a depressed fracture or intracranial haematoma, and which would otherwise have a low risk of late epilepsy. *Per contra* the importance of early epilepsy in presaging late epilepsy is less marked after injuries associated with prolonged PTA, focal

11/3   *Influence of early epilepsy on incidence of late epilepsy*

Type of injury	% LATE epilepsy				P
	No early epilepsy		After early epilepsy		
PTA $<$ 24 hours	$56/531$	11%	$25/140$	18%	<0.02
PTA $>$ 24 hours	$64/191$	34%	$32/94$	34%	NS
Depressed fracture	$80/613$	13%	$21/81$	26%	<0.01
Haematoma	$36/96$	38%	$9/32$	28%	NS
No depressed fracture or haematoma	$2/168$	1%	$23/124$	19%	<0.001
Focal signs	$58/191$	30%	$18/69$	26%	NS

11/4   *Incidence of late epilepsy after early epilepsy with different features*

Feature	% with LATE epilepsy				P
	Feature present		Feature absent		
Trivial injury	$8/32$	25%	$51/206$	25%	NS
PTA $>$ 24 hours	$32/94$	34%	$25/140$	18%	<0.01
Depressed fracture	$21/81$	26%	$21/91$	23%	NS
Haematoma	$9/32$	28%	$51/205$	25%	NS
Focal signs	$18/69$	26%	$42/170$	25%	NS
No depressed fracture or haematoma	$23/124$	27%	$36/114$	32%	NS

signs or acute intracranial haematoma and also after missile injuries; these are injuries which carry a high risk of late epilepsy whether or not early traumatic epilepsy occurs.

Once an early fit has happened other features of the injury make relatively little difference to the level of risk of late epilepsy (11/4).

11/5 *Incidence of late epilepsy after early epilepsy without depressed fracture or haematoma*

< 16 years	$^{14}/_{67}$	21%	NS
> 16 years	$^{19}/_{57}$	33%	
PTA < 24 hours	$^{15}/_{68}$	22%	NS
PTA > 24 hours	$^{16}/_{53}$	30%	
No focal signs	$^{27}/_{95}$	28%	NS
Focal signs	$^{7}/_{29}$	24%	

11/6 *LATE epilepsy after early epilepsy associated with trivial injuries*

	All cases		< 5 years		> 5 years	
Non-trivial	$^{51}/_{206}$	25%	$^{5}/_{25}$	20%	$^{46}/_{180}$	26%
Trivial	$^{8}/_{32}$	25%	$^{3}/_{17}$	18%	$^{5}/_{16}$	31%
P	NS		NS		NS	

Injuries uncomplicated by depressed fracture or haematoma were consistently associated with a high incidence of late epilepsy if there had been an early fit (11/5). And even trivial injuries, if complicated by early epilepsy, are as likely to be followed by late epilepsy as are more severe injuries, and this applied even under the age of 5 (11/6).

The form taken by the early fits does not seem to affect the risk of later epilepsy, a single fit being equally likely to be followed by late epilepsy as is repeated epilepsy or even status epilepticus (11/7); the contention of Evans that fits in the first 24 hours were not likely to be

11/7   *Number of early fits and incidence of LATE epilepsy*

One fit only	$^{24}/_{97}$	25%
Repeated fits (excluding status)	$^{31}/_{121}$	25%
Status	$^{5}/_{21}$	24%
P		NS

11/8   *Time of first early fit and incidence of late epilepsy*

Interval to early epilepsy

<1 hour	$^{21}/_{115}$	18%
1-24 hours	$^{30}/_{136}$	22%
>24 hours	$^{39}/_{156}$	25%
P		NS

11/9   *Type of early epilepsy and incidence of LATE epilepsy*

Focal early	$^{17}/_{86}$	20%
Non-focal early	$^{19}/_{61}$	31%
P		NS

11/10   *LATE epilepsy after focal early epilepsy in children*

No early epilepsy (Stöwsand < 15 years)	$^{8}/_{230}$	4%
Focal early epilepsy (Jennett <16 years)	$^{5}/_{66}$	8%
P		NS

followed by late epilepsy is not borne out (11/8). Focal early epilepsy is not so often followed by late epilepsy (11/9) and a lower recurrence rate is seen after focal early epilepsy in children. From a comparison of the present series with this characteristic and that of Stöwsand's it appears that this particular sub-division of early epilepsy may not carry a significant risk of recurrence (11/10). The other exception is "immediate epilepsy", defined as a fit occurring within moments of injury. This uncommon phenomenon consisted in the present series exclusively of a generalised fit following a mild injury in an adult; none of the small number of such patients in this series had any further epilepsy.

Chapter 12

TIME OF ONSET OF LATE EPILEPSY

There are widely varying estimates of the time after injury when patients commonly begin to have epilepsy, if they are going to develop this complication. These differences are partly explained by whether patients who have fits only in the first week, or even in the first month, are excluded or included. Also by the length of follow-up and the willingness of authors to include patients who have had a long interval between the injury and the onset of epilepsy. It is commonly stated that the majority of cases of post-traumatic epilepsy have declared themselves by the end of the first year after injury, although Symonds (1942) asserted that the prevailing view then was that the interval between trauma and injury is commonly more than a year. Which view is taken is a matter of some consequence, because on it will depend the estimate of the continuing risk of epilepsy developing for the first time at varying intervals after injury. On that will depend what advice is given to a patient about his activities, to his doctor about anticonvulsants and to his lawyer about assessing compensation or damages. Perhaps the most obvious reason why opposing views should be expressed is that about 50% of patients prove to have their first late fit within the first year, but this figure may be biased upwards by the factors already mentioned — by inclusion of early cases or by short follow-up.

Both factors must have been operating to account for Walker's (1958) finding that 75% of traumatic epilepsy had begun within three months of injury. In Gurdjian and Webster's (1958) series of 100 cases only 30% began within three months, 67% within the year. Smith *et al.* (1954) recorded 55% of 107 cases beginning within the first year, and of 43 cases of temporal lobe epilepsy reported by Vitale *et al.* (1953) 47% began in this period.

The pattern of onset after injury in the 481 patients with late epilepsy in the present study is set out in 12/1. This may be expressed graphically as the numbers which *begin* to suffer late epilepsy in each successive post-traumatic year (12/2), or as a cumulative plot of the increasing total number of patients who have had at least one fit with increasing time since injury (12/3). This series included a considerable number of patients with epilepsy beginning after 4 years and this accounts for the lower proportion of fits in the first year (56%) compared with 70% in Phillips (1954) series

12/1   *Time of first late fit in 481 with late epilepsy*

Interval after injury	Cases with onset in each period		% which have begun by end of year	
First 3 months	130	27% ⎫	1	56%
4-12 months	138	29% ⎭		
1-2 years	62	13%	2	69%
2-3 years	40	8%	3	77%
3-4 years	20	4%	4	81%
4-5 years	18	4%	5	85%
5-6 years	14	3%	6	88%
6-7 years	18	4%	7	92%
7-8 years	8	2%	8	93%
8-9 years	7	2%	9	95%
9-10 years	11	2%	10	97%
> 10 years	15	3%		

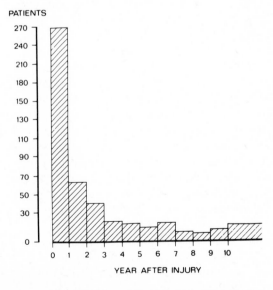

Fig. 5 (12/2). Year of first late fit in 481 patients.

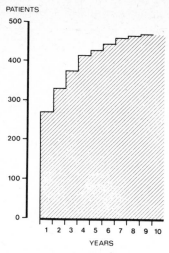

Fig. 6 (12/3). Cumulative graph showing for each year since head injury the number of patients who have developed late epilepsy.

of closed head injuries (12/4). If the analysis is restricted to the first 4 years after injury, that is to say, within a limited follow-up period, then the difference between the two series is much reduced. The inclusion within the first year figures of early fits which do not progress to late epilepsy during that year has a marked effect on the proportion of patients deemed to have traumatic epilepsy in the first year (12/5). If the calculation is then based on the first 4 years only there is now no difference between the proportion beginning in the first year in the present series and that of Phillips. Some authors have raised the possibility of a negative or a refractory period for the development of late epilepsy. If this was found by a number of different observers it might point to an aetiological factor with a certain time course. Phillips emphasised the fall off in incidence after six months, with few cases beginning epilepsy in the second year; Denny Brown made a similar observation. Phillips found the latter part of the second year particularly unusual for epilepsy to begin and so did Klotz (1955) reporting fits after leucotomy. The present series, much larger than any previous one, does not confirm such a refractory period when the months between 3 and 24 are separately analysed (12/6); the annual rate of onset indeed shows a regular decline (12/7).

Missile injuries appear to have a somewhat larger proportion occurring in the first year (75%), according to Ascroft (1941) and 73% (Russell and Whitty, 1952). In 1942 Russell stated that epilepsy rarely began more than 2-3 years after closed injuries, but that such a delay was not uncommon

12/4 *Proportion of LATE epilepsy case beginning at different times after injury*

| Total series | Onset of *LATE* epilepsy | | | |
	Phillips 145		Jennett 481	
Onset < 1 year	111	77%	268	56%
Onset 1-4 years	29	20%	122	25%
Onset > 4 years	5	3%	91	19%
Cases beginning within 4 years Onset < 1 year	$^{111}/_{140}$	79%	$^{268}/_{390}$	72%

12/5 *Time of onset of all epilepsy*

| Total | Onset of epilepsy, *including early* | | | |
	Phillips 190		Jennett 802	
Onset < 1 year	156	82%	612	76%
Onset 1-4 years	29	15%	167	13%
Onset > 4 years	5	3%	83	11%
Cases beginning within 4 years Onset < 1 year	$^{156}/_{185}$	84%	$^{612}/_{719}$	85%

after missile injuries. It seems likely that this impression may have derived from the tendency of missile injuries to be followed up for longer. Certainly, comparison of the present series, which includes many with prolonged follow-up, with that of Russell himself shows the opposite effect to that which he claimed; significantly more non-missile injuries developed epilepsy after the second year (12/8).

12/6   *Time of onset during 4-24 months*

Month of onset	Phillips 58	Jennett 91
4-6	27	34
7-9	16	7
10-12	9	26
13-15	4	6
16-18	2	4
19-24	0	14

12/7   *Time of onset within 4 years*

	Phillips 140		Jennett 390	
<3 months	59	42%	130	33%
4-12 months	52	37%	138	36%
1-2 years	6	4%	62	18%
2-3 years	15	11%	40	10%
3-4 years	8	6%	20	5%

12/8   *Time of onset of LATE epilepsy after missile and non-missile injuries*

Onset	Missile (Russell & Whitty) (excluding fits in first *month* only) 248		Non-missile (Jennett) (excluding fits in first *week* only) 408	
<1 year	181	73%	268	66%
1-2 years	46	19%	62	15%
2-5 years	21	8%	78	19%

In adults epilepsy more often developed the first year and was less often delayed beyond 4 years (12/9). This can also be observed from the cumulative percentage which have developed by the end of successive years.

Late epilepsy after more severe injuries (PTA$>$24 hours) was more likely to be delayed beyond 4 years (12/10); this tendency was more marked when a comparison was made between injuries with very brief or very prolonged PTA (12/11). When late epilepsy followed early epilepsy it was more often begun in the first year and less often after 4 years (12/12).

12/9 *Effect of age on onset of late epilepsy*

	$<$ 16 years		$>$ 16 years		P
% with onset at	131		350		
$<$ 1 year	58	44%	210	60%	$<$0.01
1-4 years	37	28%	85	24%	NS
$>$ 4 years	36	28%	55	16%	$<$0.01
% of late epilepsy series which have onset by end of	126		315		
year 1	53	42%	176	56%	$<$0.01
2	71	56%	220	70%	$<$0.01
4	90	71%	261	85%	$<$0.01

12/10 *Effect of PTA on time of onset of late epilepsy*

PTA	$<$1 year		1-4 years		$>$4 years	
$<$24 hours (221)	131	(59%)	58	(26%)	32	(15%)
$>$24 years (241)	125	(52%)	62	(26%)	54	(22%)
P	NS		NS		$<$0.05	

12/11 *Influence of very brief and very prolonged PTA on time of onset of late epilepsy*

PTA	<1 year		1-4 years		>4 years	
Nil or <1 hour (143)	89	(62%)	39	(27%)	15	(11%)
>7 days (161)	85	(53%)	34	(21%)	42	(26%)
P	NS		NS		<0.001	

12/12 *Effect of early epilepsy on time of onset of late epilepsy*

	<1 year		1-4 years		>4 years	
No early epilepsy (391)	201	(51%)	107	(27%)	83	(21%)
Early epilepsy (90)	67	(74%)	15	(17%)	8	(9%)
P	<0.001		NS		<0.001	

12/13 *Effect of depressed fracture on time of onset of late epilepsy*

	Interval to first late fit					
	<1 year		1-4 years		>4 years	
No depressed fracture (260)	168	(65%)	51	(19%)	41	(16%)
Depressed fracture (163)	76	(47%)	56	(34%)	31	(19%)
P	<0.001		<0.001		NS	

12/14 *Effect of acute haematoma on time on onset of late epilepsy*

	< 1 year		1-4 years		> 4 years	
Without acute haematoma (387)	198	(51%)	105	(27%)	84	(22%)
With acute haematoma (54)	31	(57%)	17	(32%)	6	(11%)
P	NS		NS		NS	

After depressed fractures epilepsy less often began in the first year, and more often in the 1-4 year period after injury (12/13). After acute haematoma epilepsy was rather often delayed beyond 4 years, but the difference was not significant (12/14). Focal and non-focal epilepsy had similar time patterns of onset but temporal lobe epilepsy was more often delayed beyond 4 years.

Chapter 13

TYPE OF FIT IN LATE EPILEPSY

It is more difficult to interpret the literature in respect of the type of fit than almost any other aspect of traumatic epilepsy. Series limited to missile or to blunt injury seem rarely to have been reported with this data included, whilst the way in which the terms general and focal are defined is rarely stated. Whether patients who have attacks which are focal at onset but then become generalised should be classified as having generalised or focal epilepsy is a matter of opinion. The view here is that what is most interesting is whether or not any attacks have a focal origin, although it is recognised that how often the attacks become generalised may be of more significance in terms of the disability incurred. Such large reported series as could be re-analysed using this type of classification, in which all

13/1 *Type of attack in late epilepsy*

	n	All focal	Focal only	Temporal
Mixed injuries				
Birkmayer	199	46%	13	—
Vitale	542	36%	—	19
Schou		50%	25	—
Walker and Jablon	205	65%	15	24
Missile				
Ascroft	93	—	19	
Evans	101	73	35	
Russell and Whitty	356	46	13	
Caveness	83	75	26	
Non-missile				
Phillips	142	12%		

13/2 *Type of fit in late epilepsy*

	Focal epilepsy		Temporal lobe epilepsy		
				% of total	% of focal
All ages 481	192	40%	90	19%	47%
< 16 years 131	58	44%	26	20%	45%
> 16 years 350	134	38%	64	18%	48%
P		NS		NS	

13/3 *Frequency of focal fits in late epilepsy*

Feature	Feature present		Feature absent		P
PTA > 24 hours	$98/241$	41%	$87/221$	39%	NS
Early epilepsy	$56/90$	62%	$136/391$	35%	< 0.001
Depressed fracture	$58/154$	38%	$134/327$	41%	NS
Haematoma	$31/67$	46%	$144/388$	37%	NS

patients with any attacks which have a focal component are regarded as having focal epilepsy, are set out in 13/1. In the only previous major series of non-missile injuries, only 12% of attacks had a focal component (Phillips, 1954). The mixed series averaged about 50% with a focal element, and the missile injuries up to 70%; however, in Russell and Whitty's series, confined to dural penetrating injuries, only 48% were focal. Attacks which remain focal are much less common, of the order of 20%. Only two series report temporal lobe seizures and these indicate a quarter and a fifth of patients with such seizures.

In the present series some focal feature was recognised during at least some attacks in 40% of patients and 19% had temporal lobe attacks (13/2). The proportions were similar in children and adults. Focal fits were therefore almost as frequent in this non-missile series as in reported series of missile and mixed injuries, and were much more common than reported by Phillips. The duration of PTA did not affect the type of fit nor did the presence or absence of depressed fracture, acute haematoma or previous early epilepsy (13/3).

Chapter 14

SEVERITY OF EPILEPSY

Almost as important as whether or not epilepsy occurs after injury is how likely, once it appears, it is to persist and to constitute a significant disability. Reliable data about this aspect of epilepsy is even more difficult to collect than that required to calculate incidence, because further follow-up is needed for a reasonable period after the epilepsy first appears — which, as is evident from the last chapter, can be years after the injury. It is not surprising therefore that opinions are commoner than facts, particularly in regard to non-missile injuries. However, since the first edition of this book a valuable study has been made on 356 victims of the Korean conflict, a series made up of almost equally of missile and non-missile injuries (Caveness, 1963; Weiss and Caveness, 1972). Although most of the calculations were based on the group as a whole, enough comparisons were made between the two types to indicate that there are no important differences between missile and non-missile injuries.

The two main questions of controversy are how often epilepsy ceases or remits once it has appeared, and whether there are reliable predictive criteria on which to base the prognosis of traumatic epilepsy once it has appeared. Many of the older reports refer to epilepsy having "died out" after so many years, or having "ceased", without these terms having been defined. The more experienced a clinician the less willing is he to accept that a patient is no longer liable to attacks no matter how long has passed since the last fit. In the first edition it was proposed that 2 years without a fit was perhaps a reasonable, if arbitrary, definition for remission of epilepsy. Subsequently Caveness (1963) also adopted 2 years as the criterion for cessation, pointing out that many clinicians treating adult epilepsy recommend discontinuation of anticonvulsants after two years freedom from fits; and furthermore that two years without fits is the prerequisite in many of the United States for granting a driving licence. However, in a later report (Weiss and Caveness, 1972) it was noted that of patients followed for long periods after developing traumatic epilepsy, 10% enjoyed a period of at least 2 years freedom from fits which was followed by reappearance of epilepsy. This supports the recommendation made in the first edition of this monograph that "remission" is a more suitable term to use than "cessation".

The only meaningful way of assessing the severity of epilepsy is by the number of attacks in unit time. It is obvious that certain types of attack are less disabling than others, for example minor temporal lobe fits which are scarcely noticeable, or attacks which occur only at night. Some authors (e.g. Russell and Davies-Jones, 1969) have sought to take account of this by quoting the number of grand mal attacks in unit time; so many patients have different types of attacks at different times that this seems an unwise and artificial distinction. Therefore the rule here has been, as in most other studies, to regard fits of any kind as being of significance.

Certain problems arise in assessing severity and remission. One is whether or not early fits are included. It has been established (Chapter 11) that two thirds or more with early epilepsy do not have any further fits after the first week. Their inclusion will therefore reduce the overall severity in the series, and will increase the remission rate. Another is whether fit frequency is calculated on an average rate per annum, or the number in the last year of follow-up, or the total number since injury. This leads to another question, the duration of follow-up. This is commonly defined as so many years since injury, but when assessing severity and remission rate enough time must elapse after the development of epilepsy for the frequency of seizures to be estimated, and for remission to occur. If, for example, a patient in a series followed for 5 years after injury should have a fit in the last few weeks of that period it is misleading to include him in the group with very infrequent seizures, on the basis that only one fit has occurred in 5 years; this may prove to have been the first of a frequently recurring series of fits. For these reasons all the data about severity of late epilepsy in the present study is based on patients followed for at least 2 years after the onset of late epilepsy.

With these cautions in mind the significant literature on this topic can now be reviewed, remembering that in many instances sufficient information was not available to enable the reader to discern what conditions applied in a given reported series (e.g. whether or not early epilepsy was included, the duration of follow-up and so on).

Ascroft (1941), reporting 74 missile injuries with epilepsy beginning after 3 months found that every one of 16 patients who enjoyed a remission of at least 5 years had begun to suffer epilepsy before the end of the 2nd year after injury. This view that the later epilepsy develops the more likely it is to persist was subsequently confirmed for non-missile injuries by Phillips (1954), and also in Caveness' mixed group of combat injuries.

In a group of 199 mixed, closed and open injuries Birkmayer (1949) found 53% with one to six fits per annum, 29% with 7-12, and 18% with more than one fit per month. Smith *et al.* (1954) reviewed over 500 mixed injuries compiled from German welfare records and found 40% with less than one fit a month but 25% had up to 3 fits a month. Russell and Whitty (1952) assessed the frequency of fits in 279 penetrating missile injuries (dura torn) found that 47% had less than 5 fits in the first 5 years since injury; only 34% had more than 2 fits per year. However, in a later report on 195 men from the same series, followed for 15-25 years, Russell and Davies-Jones (1969) reported that 25% were still having major fits and that 5% were suffering from more than 6 grand mal attacks per year.

In Walker's (1956) series of 246 missile injuries with epilepsy, reviewed 10 years after injury, 46% had had no fits for several years. Between the 5th and 10th years 25% had no epilepsy and 18% had only 1-2 fits per year. He concluded that epilepsy tends to disappear after 5 years or so, and that after a year's freedom from epilepsy in the first five years there was a 40% chance that no further epilepsy would occur in the next 5 to 8 years. In a discussion following this paper Penfield challenged this as being over-optimistic; but Walker asserted that he considered Penfield's pessimism to be unjustified, viz "when an objective lesion of the brain can be demonstrated permanent disappearance of attacks never occurs" (Penfield and Erikson, 1941).

14/1 *Frequency of fits after different injuries* (Caveness, 1963)

	Missile 83		Non-missile 26		P
1-3 fits	26	31%	13	50%	NS
4-30 fits	29	35%	3	12%	NS
Multiple	28	34%	10	39%	NS
Later ceased	48	52%	15	58%	NS

14/2 *Effect of fit frequency on subsequent cessation of late epilepsy* (mixed missile and non-missile, Caveness, 1963)

Fit frequency	Proportion ceased		
1-3	$33/39$	85%	$P < 0.01$
4-30	$17/32$	55%	
Multiple	$8/38$	21%	$P < 0.01$

14/3 *Number of initial late fits and severity*
(derived from Weiss and Caveness, 1972)

Severity	In first 6 months			
	One fit		≥2 fits		P
Persisted 4 years	10/32	31%	16/23	70%	<0.01
Persisted 8 years	13/20	43%	13/22	59%	NS
Multiple fits	4/27	15%	15/28	54%	<0.01

Severity	In first year				
	One fit		2 fits		≥3 fits	P (<3 v ≥3 fits)
Persisted 4 years	3/22	14%	8/16	50%	30/35	86%	<0.001
Persisted 8 years	6/20	30%	5/15	33%	23/35	66%	<0.01
Multiple fits	2/22	9%	6/18	33%	22/33	67%	<0.001

14/4 *Severity of late epilepsy*

Age	n	>1 fit/month	<1 fit/month >1 fit/6 months	<1 fit/6 months	Remission
All ages	328	118 36%	69 21%	60 18%	81 25%
<16 years	98	42 43%	12 12%	17 17%	27 28%
>16 years	230	76 35%	57 25%	43 19%	54 23%
P		NS	<0.02	NS	NS
<5 years	29	13 45%	0	6 21%	10 34%
>5 years	299	105 35%	69 23%	54 18%	71 24%
P		NS	<0.01	NS	NS

14/5   *Effect of time of onset on severity of late epilepsy*

First late fit	More than 1 fit per month		Remission	
< 4 years (261)	84	32%	77	30%
> 4 years (68)	34	50%	4	6%
P	< 0.01		< 0.001	

14/6   (a) *Cessation of late epilepsy*
(Caveness, 1963)

Onset < 2 years	$^{54}/_{95}$	57%
Onset > 2 years	$^{4}/_{14}$	29%
P		NS

(b) *Persistence of late epilepsy*
(Weiss and Caveness, 1972)

Onset 1 week-6 months	$^{19}/_{29}$	66%
Onset 6 months-1 year	$^{13}/_{18}$	72%
P		NS

The analysis carried out on 356 Korean combat victims by Caveness provides the best basis for comparison with the present study. In the first paper (Caveness, 1963) the emphasis was on *cessation* (more than 2 years without a fit); in the second (Weiss and Caveness, 1972) it was on *persistence*, which, although not precisely defined, would appear to indicate the opposite of cessation. Thus the cessation rate in 1963 was 53% and in 1972 the persistence rate was 56% at 4 years and 47% at 8 years. Frequency of fits was described as 1-3 or 4-30 fits and "multiple" (too many to count), although it was not clear what time period this covered. No difference was found between the missile and non-missile injuries for the proportions with multiple fits or with cessation (14/1). When fits occurred frequently they seldom ceased (14/2).

This was expressed differently in the 1972 paper, where persistence and the occurrence of multiple fits were related to the number of late fits occurring in the first 6 months or the first year after injury. Two thirds of those who had 3 or more fits in the first year continued to have multiple fits and two thirds were still suffering from epilepsy 8 years after injury (14/3).

In the present series the number with frequent fits (36%) was very similar to that reported by Caveness (35%); but the remission rate (25%) was half that of Caveness (14/4). The severity of epilepsy was similar in children under 5, and there was no difference between children as a whole and adults. When epilepsy was delayed beyond 4 years there was a greater likelihood of fits, and significantly less chance of remission (14/5); there was no difference between fits coming on within 3 months, in the 4-12 month period or the 1-4 year period after injury — only at 4 years was a significant change observed. This confirmed the observations of Ascroft, of Phillips and of Caveness, that epilepsy that is delayed on onset is more likely to persist. Cessation was significantly less frequent when epilepsy began after 2 years in Caveness' series (14/6a); persistence was similar for epilepsy beginning between one week and 6 months and between 6 and 12 months (14/6b).

14/7 *Severity with different types of late fit*

	More than one fit per month		Remission	
Focal 132	48	38%	29	22%
Non-focal 197	70	38%	52	26%
P	NS		NS	
Temporal lobe 71	32	45%	7	10%
Other types 258	86	33%	74	29%
P	NS		< 0.001	

14/8 *Severity with different types of late fit*

Type of fit	Cessation of late epilepsy (Caveness, 1963)		Severity of late epilepsy (Weiss and Caveness, 1972)			
			Persisting 4 years		Multiple fits	
Focal	$^{38}/_{77}$	49%	$^{47}/_{76}$	62%	$^{28}/_{75}$	37%
Non-focal	$^{20}/_{32}$	63%	$^{9}/_{24}$	38%	$^{1}/_{25}$	4%
P	NS		< 0.05		< 0.01	

No difference was observed in the present series between focal and non-focal attacks in respect of frequent fits or of remission (14/7), but temporal lobe epilepsy was less likely to remit. This is at variance with Weiss and Caveness' finding that focal epilepsy was both more likely to be frequent and to persist (14/8). Frequent fits were rather less common after injuries associated with depressed fracture, intracranial haematoma or early epilepsy, but more common when PTA exceeded 24 hours (14/9a). Remission rate was more common after early epilepsy or haematoma, less common after prolonged PTA, and was unaffected by depressed fracture (14/9b).

The nature of early epilepsy affected the severity of late epilepsy in Caveness' series, single and non-focal early fits being associated with a somewhat lower incidence of multiple late fits, and of persistence at 4 years (14/10). These trends were even less marked in the present series, but after focal early epilepsy late epilepsy more often took the form of multiple late fits and more often persisted than after non-focal early fits. In Caveness' series several other factors had no effect at all on fit frequency or remission rate — duration of coma, dural penetration, depth of brain wound and severity of immediate complications (haemorrhage and infection).

In conclusion, it would appear that it is unwise to be over-optimistic about expecting epilepsy to go into permanent remission. There is no doubt that many patients suffer only occasional attacks, and that prolonged remission of epilepsy is by no means uncommon. Moreover it is likely that more efficient follow-up is achieved in patients who continue to suffer seizures, in that they are likely to remain under hospital supervision.

14/9 *Severity of late epilepsy after injuries with different features*

	% with more than one fit per month			
Feature	Feature present		Feature absent	P
PTA > 24 hours	$^{65}/_{164}$ 40%		$^{43}/_{148}$ 29%	< 0.05
Early epilepsy	$^{17}/_{59}$ 29%		$^{101}/_{269}$ 38%	NS
Depressed fracture	$^{37}/_{126}$ 29%		$^{58}/_{158}$ 37%	NS
Haematoma	$^{15}/_{53}$ 28%		$^{103}/_{275}$ 37%	NS

	% with remission			
Feature	Feature present		Feature absent	P
PTA > 24 hours	$^{34}/_{164}$ 21%		$^{44}/_{148}$ 30%	NS
Early epilepsy	$^{22}/_{59}$ 37%		$^{59}/_{269}$ 22%	< 0.02
Depressed fracture	$^{37}/_{126}$ 29%		$^{43}/_{158}$ 27%	NS
Haematoma	$^{20}/_{53}$ 38%		$^{61}/_{175}$ 22%	< 0.02

14/10 *Character of early epilepsy and severity of late*
(Weiss and Caveness, 1972)

	Persisted 4 years		Multiple fits	
Single early fit	$^{3}/_{17}$	18%	$^{4}/_{17}$	24%
Repeated early fits	$^{4}/_{9}$	44%	$^{3}/_{9}$	33%
P		NS		NS
Focal early	$^{7}/_{20}$	35%	$^{3}/_{20}$	15%
Non-focal early	$^{1}/_{6}$	17%	$^{0}/_{6}$	0
P		NS		NS

Nonetheless the present series, together with the careful studies of Caveness, indicate that late traumatic epilepsy is as likely to persist as not, and to do so for many years. The concept that epilepsy represents a passing stage in the healing process after head injury, and is therefore likely to be temporary, proves to be founded more on fancy than on fact.

Chapter 15

INCIDENCE OF LATE EPILEPSY

The frequency of late epilepsy after combat missile injuries has shown a remarkable consistency through several wars, the rate being higher when the dura is penetrated (15/1). Military populations are homogeneous and the machinery for good documentation and reliable follow-up is at hand. The only cause for surprise, and for disappointment, is that the greatly reduced infection rate in recent times should have had no obvious effect on the incidence of late epilepsy. There may be a balancing effect, in that improved methods of resuscitation and treatment may be securing the survival of men so seriously injured that they would previously have died, and that the survivors from such injuries compensate for the infected cases no longer seen, by contributing a high epilepsy rate. If so, the balancing has been remarkably finely adjusted.

Apart from dural penetration few factors seem to affect the incidence; Russell and Whitty found epilepsy more often with wounds near the central sulcus, and less often with damage within 5 cm of the sagittal sinus. More extensive wounds, as indicated by the depth of penetration or the occurrence of hemiplegia, had only a slightly increased incidence of epilepsy. A number of series, particularly of combat injuries, are made up of missile and non-missile injuries which are not always separately analysed; nonetheless such series are of considerable size and are often quoted (15/2).

Estimates of the incidence of epilepsy after closed, civilian or non-missile injuries vary widely and there is seldom certainty about either the criteria required for entry to the series or about the duration of the follow-up. The finding that late epilepsy after non-missile injury is delayed beyond the first year in almost half the cases, and beyond the fourth year in a quarter, indicates that rates are bound to vary with duration of follow-up. Reichmann (1927) quoted 0.5% for injuries with skull fracture, and less for those without, and stated that epilepsy was a rare complication of peace-time. Malling (1953), discussing this paper, agreed that epilepsy was indeed a rarity; he claimed to know of only two cases, out of many thousands of head injuries, who had developed chronic epilepsy with a certain probability that it was due to head injury. Here lies one explanation for these very low estimates, in that only persisting

15/1 *Late epilepsy after missile injuries*

	World War I	World War II		Korea
	Ascroft (316)	Walker (295)	Russell (820)	Caveness (211)
All cases	35%	34%	–	35%
Dura intact	22%	–	–	24%
Dura penetrated	41%	–	43%	42%

15/2 *Mixed war series*

	Credner		Walker		Caveness	
All	38%	(1990)	28%	(739)	31%	(356)
Dura intact	19%	(756)	14%	(267)	20%	(226)
Dura torn	50%	(1234)	36%	(472)	50%	(130)

(Data from Caveness W. F., Walker, A.E. and Ascroft, P.B., 1962)

epilepsy was being acknowledged. Nevertheless Denny-Brown (1943) considered that the best estimate available, because it was from a large and unselected population, was that of Feinberg (1934). In 47,130 head injuries, seen for insurance purposes in Switzerland, he reported 0.1% with epilepsy in the whole series and 0.5% for those with skull fractures. However, another insurance series of 200 cases yielded 5% with epilepsy (Schou, 1933). Rowbotham (1949) and Wilson (1955) each quoted 2.6% with epilepsy in 430 civilian injuries followed for 5 years, and in 600 concussions, respectively. In Phillips' report of 6% in 500 non-missile injuries in servicemen neither early fits nor patients with previous epilepsy were excluded and the follow-up was for only 2-3 years.

The non-missile cases in the combat series of Walker and Jablon (1947) and of Caveness and Liss (1961) had considerably higher epilepsy rates — 24% of 444 and 12% of 196 respectively; but in Evans (1962) series of 149 it was only 8%. The figure of Walker approaches that given by Freeman (1953) for the incidence of epilepsy after leucotomy (26%), which was

15/3   *Effect of injury site on incidence of LATE epilepsy*

| | Missile | | Non-missile |
	Dura intact	Dura torn	(Dura intact)
Parietal	$13/27$ 48%	$23/31$ 74%	$6/18$ 33%
Other	$7/45$ 16%	$40/94$ 43%	$18/136$ 13%
P	<0.01	<0.01	NS

(Data from Caveness, 1963)

confirmed by Klotz (1955) who stressed the increased incidence associated with bilateral operations; leucotomy can be regarded as an example of simple cortical contusion without concussion.

Caveness (1963) explored factors associated with increased risk of epilepsy. In both missile and non-missile injuries parietal lobe injuries were significantly more frequently followed by epilepsy; this held for missile injuries whether dura was intact or torn; but there were too few non-missile injuries with dura torn for comparison (15/3).

The Present Series

To assess the overall incidence of late epilepsy by following up large numbers of head injuries, many of them mildly injured, would be difficult if not impossible. Early on in the study it was evident that the incidence varied widely according to the type of injury, and further elaboration of this investigation has confirmed that there are three main factors which significantly increase the risk of late epilepsy − namely early epilepsy, depressed fracture and acute intracranial haematoma (15/4). Each of these factors is examined in detail in separate chapters whilst the validity of the follow-up series as a whole, and the means whereby representative series without these complications were derived, has been discussed in Chapter 6. Apart from these three main factors two issues remain to be discussed, the influence of age and the significance of duration of PTA, particularly in patients without the three main complications.

The age at injury of the patients with late epilepsy was similar to that of the Oxford series of head injuries (15/5). However, in those followed the incidence of epilepsy is higher in adults than in children as a whole (under 16 years); but for patients under and over 5 years of age there was no difference in the epilepsy rate (15/6).

15/4 *Incidence of late epilepsy after different features of injury*

Feature	P (present v Oxford)	Feature *absent* Oxford follow-up		Feature *present*		Feature *absent* by extrapolation		P (present v extrapolated)
Early epilepsy	<0.001	$^{18}/_{240}$	8%	$^{59}/_{238}$	28%	$^{29}/_{868}$	3%	<0.001
Depressed fracture	<0.01	$^{17}/_{223}$	8%	$^{100}/_{693}$	14%	$^{27}/_{832}$	3%	<0.001
Acute haematoma	<0.001	$^{18}/_{240}$	8%	$^{45}/_{128}$	35%	$^{27}/_{868}$	3%	<0.001

15/5 *Age at injury of unselected survivors and late epilepsy series*

	< 5 years		5-15 years		> 16 years	
Oxford series (896)	75	(8%)	122	(14%)	619	(78%)
Late epilepsy (481)	40	(8%)	91	(19%)	350	(73%)

15/6 *Effect of age on incidence of late epilepsy*

< 5 years	$24/149$	16%
5-15 years	$30/293$	10%
>16 years	$131/539$	24%

< 5 years	$24/149$	16%		< 16 years	$54/442$	12%
> 5 years	$161/832$	19%		>16 years	$131/539$	24%
P		NS		P		< 0.001

15/7 *Effect of PTA on incidence of late epilepsy*

	PTA < 24 hours		PTA > 24 hours		P
All ages	$81/671$	12%	$96/285$	34%	< 0.001
< 5 years	$15/121$	12%	$7/23$	30%	< 0.05
> 5 years	$66/550$	12%	$89/262$	34%	< 0.001
< 16 years	$30/350$	9%	$19/82$	23%	< 0.001
> 16 years	$51/321$	16%	$77/203$	38%	< 0.001

Late epilepsy was twice as common in patients with more than 24 hours PTA and this applied to both adults and children, including the under 5's (15/7). This association between prolonged PTA and late epilepsy is confirmed by the finding that patients with more than 24 hours PTA formed only 17% of the unselected Oxford survivors but accounted for 52% of the late epilepsy series (15/8). There was no difference between the proportion of patients with no amnesia, in the head injury series and the late epilepsy series.

The influence of prolonged PTA was observed only in patients suffering from injuries already associated with an increased risk of epilepsy (15/9). The interaction between PTA and these factors is explored in the chapters dealing with early epilepsy (pages 64, 5), with depressed fracture (page 97)

15/8 *PTA of unselected survivors and late epilepsy series*

PTA	Oxford survivors (883)		Late epilepsy (453)		P
Nil	108	12%	56	12%	NS
<1 hour	414	47%	87	19%	<0.001
1-24 hours	207	24%	73	16%	<0.01
1-7 days	64	7%	76	17%	<0.001
>7 days	90	10%	161	36%	<0.001
<24 hours	729	83%	216	48%	<0.001
>24 hours	154	17%	237	52%	<0.001

15/9 *Effect of PTA on incidence of late epilepsy after different types of injury*

	PTA < 24 hours		PTA > 24 hours		P
Early epilepsy	$25/140$	18%	$32/94$	34%	<0.01
Depressed fracture	$45/520$	9%	$53/166$	32%	<0.01
Haematoma	$12/47$	26%	$33/79$	42%	NS
None of these	$1/100$	1%	$1/68$	1.5%	NS

and acute haematoma (page 136). After injuries not associated with local damage, that is to say without depressed fracture or haematoma, the duration of PTA made little difference to the incidence of late epilepsy; in these injuries the most important criterion was whether or not early epilepsy had occurred (15/10). When such injuries were not complicated by early epilepsy it was exceptional for late epilepsy to occur, even when PTA had been prolonged. By extrapolation from the Oxford 1,000 series, in which milder injuries were so common and early epilepsy occurred in only 5%, it is possible to calculate the incidence of late epilepsy after an unselected series of injuries without depressed fracture or haematoma. This is 2% for the whole series, but is significantly commoner when PTA exceeds 24 hours.

15/10 *Effect of late epilepsy after injuries without depressed fracture or haematoma*

	PTA < 24 hours		PTA > 24 hours		P
After early epilepsy	$^{15}/_{68}$	22%	$^{16}/_{53}$	30%	NS
No early epilepsy	$^{1}/_{100}$	1%	$^{1}/_{68}$	1.5%	NS
P	< 0.001		< 0.001		
Unselected injuries (by extrapolation from Oxford 1000)	$^{9}/_{661}$	1%	$^{5}/_{112}$	5%	< 0.05

Overall Incidence of Late Epilepsy

It is now possible to calculate the overall incidence of epilepsy using the Oxford series as an unselected head injury series, and applying to each sub-group within it the appropriate epilepsy rate as indicated by this study. Such a calculation gives the number of cases of epilepsy which would be expected if all cases were followed; the overall figure is about 5% developing epilepsy, on the basis of 4 years minimum follow-up. This is an abstraction of limited practical use, because any doctor concerned to estimate the risk in a given case will presumably always have some details about the injury, which will enable the patient to be placed in one of the sub-groups for which more accurate estimates of risk are available. The

15/11   *Frequency of positive family history*

	No late epilepsy		With late epilepsy		P
All cases	$^{11}/_{271}$	4%	$^{9}/_{95}$	10%	NS
<16 years	$^{8}/_{155}$	5%	$^{5}/_{29}$	17%	<0.02
>16 years	$^{3}/_{116}$	3%	$^{4}/_{66}$	6%	NS

reduction of this risk with the passage of time, provided that no epilepsy has developed, is the subject of a separate chapter. A positive family history was more common in patients who developed late epilepsy, but significantly so only in children (15/11).

Chapter 16

DEPRESSED FRACTURE

The single consistent strand which runs through the confused and conflicting literature of traumatic epilepsy is the assertion that depressed fracture of the skull is an important predisposing factor. Indeed it was predicted over 60 years ago (English, 1906) that once elevation of depressed fracture became routine traumatic epilepsy would become a rarity. That author found six of seven patients with focal epilepsy due to trauma had a depressed fracture. Half a century later a similar view was expressed by Mock (1950), that cases of traumatic epilepsy are usually associated with depressed fractures. The present study indicates that depressed fracture in fact accounts for only about one case of traumatic epilepsy in five, both in the first week and later.

Estimates of the frequency of epilepsy after depressed fracture vary widely. Neither of two reports which quoted quite high figures (Evans 25%, Phillips 68%) separated early from late epilepsy. However, since the original reports from the present study there have been several series reporting the incidence of early epilepsy, which range from 5-12%; the only other figure for late epilepsy is 10% (16/1).

A series of 1,000 depressed fractures has now been analysed, from Glasgow, Oxford and Rotterdam. The close resemblance between depressed fractures in the unselected Oxford series and those subsequently collected has been shown (6/3, p. 19); and also between fractures in these three cities (Fig. 1, page 19) no serious doubt can remain that a valid sample of depressed fractures, as seen in Western Europe, has been studied.

A fracture was deemed to be depressed if the inner table was indented by more than the thickness of the skull. Puncture of the skull by sharp instruments, such as scissors, knitting needles and nails, were included but high velocity missile injuries and birth injuries were excluded. A basal fracture involving the air sinuses was not regarded as a depressed fracture unless there was also depression of the vault. The term *closed* fracture indicates no overlying scalp laceration; *compound* injury implies a scalp laceration and includes both those with intact dura and with torn dura; the word "penetrating" is avoided because of ambiguity as to whether the skin, the scalp or the dura was involved. It is natural to speculate how closely a depressed fracture resembles a missile injury. Indeed it was the presence of so many depressed fractures in the present series which led to

97

16/1   Epilepsy after depressed fracture

Early epilepsy

White and Mixter	(1948)	$6/54$	11%
Stöwsand and Giele	(1966)	$15/122$	12%
Hendrick and Harris	(1968)	$30/300$	10%
Carbraal and Abeysuriya	(1969)	$30+/310$	10-12%
Jamieson and Yelland	(1972)	$16/322$	5%

Late epilepsy

Stöwsand and Giele	(1966)	$8/77$	10%

a change of title for this monograph from "blunt" injuries to "non-missile" injuries. Certainly penetration of the skull by low velocity shell fragments is likely to produce very similar brain damage to a puncture wound due to a fragment of wrecked car or even that dealt by a sharp weapon such as a screwdriver or a nail. In both instances brain damage is likely to be localised, consciousness is lost briefly if at all, and whether any focal signs appear depends largely on the site of wounding. In more severe injuries the difference may be greater; though in both instances there is likely to be more widespread brain damage, after missile injuries this is due to the greater amount of local destruction, whilst after non-missile injuries it is due to diffuse effects of acceleration-deceleration forces. In this respect it is of interest to notice that missile injuries with the dura intact show a higher epilepsy rate than do similar non-missile injuries (Caveness, 1963).

The importance of dural penetration was once believed to lie in the risk of infection with the concomitant likelihood of more extensive scarring. The failure of the epilepsy rate to fall with the progressive reduction in infection rate in successive wars (15/1 and 15/2, see p. 90) suggests that this factor is less significant than was once believed. Certainly there are occasional instances of epilepsy associated with infective complications, particularly in the first week, but it seems likely that the real significance of dural penetration is that it usually indicates more extensive cortical damage. This too seems likely to be the essential difference between missile and non-missile injuries when taken as a whole, namely that cortical damage is usually more marked after missile injury.

Clinical Characteristics of Civilian Depressed Fracture

Half the patients were under the age of 16 years, a third of these being under 5. Because the brain damage is localised prolonged amnesia was unusual, less than a quarter having more than 24 hours PTA; less than half had been unconscious for more than a few minutes. Almost half of all depressed fractures, both in adults and in children, were due to road accidents. In adults the next commonest cause was injury at work, and assault was also quite common event (16/2). In children accidents around the home and in the course of sport were common.

Classification of site may be by the bones of the skull, or the lobes of the brain, although published reports do not always declare clearly which has been employed. The present series as a whole (information available for 911 cases) was initially classified only into frontal, temporo-parietal, and occipital *bone* involvement. However, in order to make a more detailed study, and to allow comparison with published figures for missile series analysed by *lobes* of the brain, a subset of 300 cases for which radiographs were still available was examined. It was established that this "detailed" series was a valid sample of the "total" series, in particular that the overall incidence of early and of late epilepsy was similar. Analysis by lobes of the brain was based on a chart published by Russell (1947) for missile injuries, and which appears to have been the basis also of subsequently published series of missile injuries from Ascroft (Caveness, Walker and Ascroft, 1962) and from Caveness (1963) — in so far as these

16/2   *Causes of depressed fractures*

	< 16 years (444)		> 16 years (495)	
Road accident	221	50%	219	44%
Work	6	1%	142	29%
Assault	18	4%	76	15%
Home	144	35%	40	8%
Sport	55	12%	18	4%

16/3   *Frequency of fractures in different sites by lobes of brain*

		Missile (Russell and Whitty)		Non-missile (Detailed series)	
A	Pre-frontal and inferior frontal	160	27%	88	29%
B	Motor and premotor	127	21%	92	30%
C	Parietal lobe	170	28%	67	23%
D	Temporal lobe	71	12%	6	2%
E	Occipital lobe	73	12%	47	16%

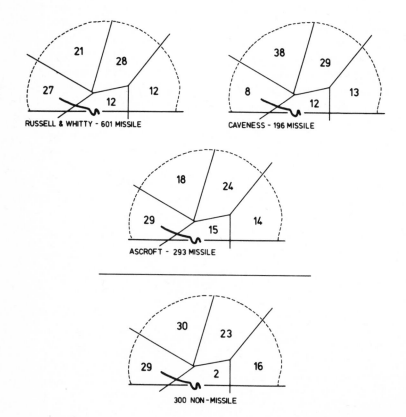

Fig. 7. Distribution of fractures by lobes of the brain (as % of series each site).

authors employed the same descriptive terms. The distribution of fractures by lobes was similar for the three missile series; in the non-missile series temporal fractures were distinctly rare, and frontal lobe fractures more common than with missile injuries (16/3). When the analysis is by *bones* (16/4) the proportion labelled as frontal drops from 59% to 39%, which emphasises the need to be clear as to which method of description is being used.

Early Epilepsy

Incidence

One or more fits occurred in the first week after injury in 10% of patients with depressed fracture, more than twice the incidence after other injuries (16/5). Depressed fracture increased the incidence of early

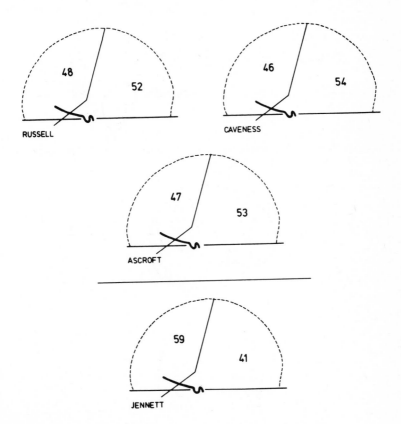

Fig. 8. Relation of fractures to Rolandic (central) sulcus.

16/4   *Frequency of fractures in different sites by bones of skull*

	Total series 911		Detailed series 300	
Frontal bone	386	42%	118	39%
Temporo-parietal	453	50%	164	55%
			(Temporal 6	2%)
Occipital	72	8%	18	6%

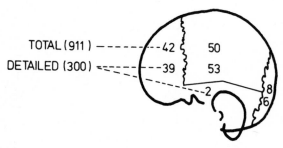

Fig. 9. Distribution of non-missile fractures by bone involved (as % of each series).

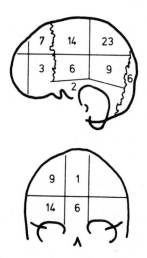

Fig. 10. More detailed analysis of site (as % of detailed series).

epilepsy both in children and in adults; but after injuries associated with prolonged PTA or focal signs the already increased rate of early epilepsy was not further accentuated by a depressed fracture.

The epilepsy rate after depressed fracture was similar whatever the other features of the injury (16/6) — the duration of PTA, the presence of focal signs or the age of the patient, whether the fracture was closed or compound and in the latter case whether the dura was intact or not. The site of fracture likewise had little effect although occipital fractures, which

16/5   *Effect of depressed fracture on incidence of early epilepsy*

Feature	No depressed fracture		Depressed fracture		P
All	$^{37}/_{912}$	4%	$^{96}/_{947}$	10%	<0.001
<16 years	$^{9}/_{170}$	5%	$^{49}/_{459}$	11%	<0.05
>16 years	$^{28}/_{735}$	4%	$^{47}/_{488}$	10%	<0.001
<24 hours PTA	$^{16}/_{683}$	2%	$^{65}/_{697}$	9%	<0.001
>24 hours PTA	$^{14}/_{137}$	10%	$^{27}/_{230}$	12%	NS
No focal signs	$^{8}/_{663}$	1%	$^{71}/_{756}$	9%	<0.001
Focal signs	$^{22}/_{169}$	15%	$^{25}/_{192}$	13%	NS

16/6   *Incidence of early epilepsy after depressed fracture with various features*

Feature	Feature present		Feature absent		P
<5 years	$^{11}/_{138}$	8%	$^{82}/_{783}$	11%	NS
<16 years	$^{49}/_{459}$	11%	$^{47}/_{488}$	10%	NS
PTA >24 hours	$^{27}/_{230}$	12%	$^{69}/_{697}$	9%	NS
Focal signs	$^{25}/_{192}$	13%	$^{71}/_{756}$	9%	NS
Compound	$^{82}/_{840}$	10%	$^{4}/_{107}$	13%	NS
Dura torn	$^{47}/_{419}$	11%	$^{35}/_{421}$	8%	NS

16/7   *Effect of site of depressed fracture on incidence of early epilepsy*

			P
1. *By bones of skull*			
Frontal bone	$^{41}/_{386}$	11%	
Temporo-parietal	$^{49}/_{453}$	11%	NS
Occipital	$^{3}/_{72}$	4%	
2. *By lobes of brain*			
Frontal lobe	$^{25}/_{180}$	14%	NS
Other lobes	$^{9}/_{120}$	8%	

are uncommon, were less often followed by early epilepsy; but there was no significant difference between fractures of the frontal and temporo-parietal *bones* (16/7). When these are regrouped to correspond with the *lobes* of the brain there is a somewhat higher incidence with frontal wounds (14%) than after those posterior to the central sulcus (8%).

Character of Early Epilepsy

Almost 75% of the patients with early epilepsy after depressed fracture had their first (or only) fit within 24 hours of injury; more than half of these occurred in the first hour. There were significantly more very early fits than after injuries without depressed fracture (16/8). An even higher proportion of fits were in the first hour when PTA was less than 24 hours, whilst after prolonged PTA the first fit was more often delayed beyond 24 hours (16/9). This reflects the influence of PTA on the interval to the

16/8   *Effect of depressed fracture on interval to first fit*

	First hour		1-24 hours		> 24 hours	
No depressed fracture (282)	69	25%	95	34%	118	42%
After depressed fracture (100)	39	39%	33	33%	28	28%
P	< 0.01		NS		< 0.02	

16/9 *Effect of PTA on interval to first fit after depressed fracture*

	First hour		1-24 hours		> 24 hours	
PTA < 24 (65)	31	48%	19	29%	15	23%
PTA > 24 (30)	6	20%	12	40%	12	40%
P	< 0.02		NS		NS	

16/10 *Type of early fit*

	Any focal type		Focal motor only	
No depressed fracture (286)	164	57%	121	43%
After depressed fracture (100)	56	56%	44	44%
P	NS		NS	

16/11 *Effect of PTA on proportion of patients with early fits which are focal*

			P
(a) PTA < 24 hours	$^{36}/_{65}$	55%	NS
PTA > 24 hours	$^{18}/_{31}$	58%	
(b) PTA < 1 hour	$^{27}/_{46}$	59%	NS
PTA > 1 hour	$^{17}/_{40}$	43%	

first fit in the whole series of patients with early epilepsy (10/6). Contrary to what might be expected, considering that the brain damage was so often focal, neither focal fits (of any kind) nor focal motor attacks were more common after depressed fractures than after other types of injury (16/10). There was no difference in this proportion whether PTA was greater or less

16/12 *Effect of depressed fracture on number of early fits*

	Single fit		Status	
No depressed fracture (280)	82	29%	33	12%
Depressed fracture (99)	52	52%	7	7%
P	<0.001		NS	

than 24 hours (16/11) but when PTA was less than 1 hour the proportion of focal fits was somewhat higher, although not significantly so. Half the patients with early epilepsy after depressed fractures had only a single fit, a significantly higher proportion than after other injuries (16/12).

Late Epilepsy

More than three quarters of the series were followed for at least a year, and it was confirmed that these were a valid sample of the original series (6/6, page 21).

After depressed fracture late epilepsy was significantly more frequent, but this difference was much less marked in children (16/13). Comparison

16/13 *Effect of depressed fracture on incidence of late epilepsy*

	All ages
No depressed fracture	$27/832$ 3%
Depressed fracture	$104/694$ 15%
P	<0.001

	<16 years		>16 years	
No depressed fracture	$10/174$	6%	$20/658$	3%
Depressed fracture	$31/345$	9%	$69/348$	20%
P	NS		<0.001	

with the epilepsy rate in patients with depressed fractures sustained at different ages revealed no difference between those under and over 5 years but epilepsy was significantly more common over the age of 16 (16/14). In the original series adults had a higher proportion with long PTA, with focal signs or with dural tearing, features which are associated with an increased risk of epilepsy (16/15), whilst this certainly contributed to the higher incidence of epilepsy in adults, this was evident after depressed fractures associated with a wide range of different conditions (16/16). Hendrick and Harris (1968) reported a low incidence of late epilepsy after depressed fractures in children, although it was not clear how many of their cases had been followed.

16/14 *Incidence of late epilepsy after depressed fracture at different ages*

			P
<5 years	$^{13}/_{109}$	12%	NS
5-16 years	$^{18}/_{236}$	8%	< 0.001
>16 years	$^{69}/_{348}$	20%	
<5 years	$^{13}/_{109}$	12%	NS
>5 years	$^{87}/_{584}$	15%	
<16 years	$^{31}/_{345}$	9%	<0.001
>16 years	$^{69}/_{348}$	20%	

16/15 *Association of various features with age at injury*

Feature	All ages		<16 years		>16 years		P
PTA > 24 hours	$^{230}/_{928}$	25%	$^{72}/_{449}$	16%	$^{158}/_{479}$	33%	<0.001
Focal signs	$^{192}/_{928}$	20%	$^{68}/_{449}$	15%	$^{124}/_{479}$	26%	<0.001
Compound	$^{840}/_{947}$	89%	$^{393}/_{459}$	86%	$^{448}/_{489}$	92%	<0.01
Dura torn (in compound)	$^{420}/_{840}$	50%	$^{176}/_{393}$	45%	$^{244}/_{448}$	55%	<0.01

16/16   *Incidence of late epilepsy in children and adults with different features*

Feature	< 16 years		> 16 years		P
PTA < 24 hours	$^{14}/_{286}$	5%	$^{32}/_{234}$	14%	<0.001
PTA > 24 hours	$^{15}/_{54}$	28%	$^{38}/_{112}$	34%	NS
No focal signs	$^{20}/_{287}$	7%	$^{42}/_{259}$	16%	<0.001
With focal signs	$^{11}/_{58}$	19%	$^{29}/_{90}$	31%	NS
No early epilepsy	$^{27}/_{304}$	9%	$^{52}/_{308}$	17%	<0.01
After early epilepsy	$^{4}/_{41}$	10%	$^{17}/_{40}$	43%	<0.001
Dura intact	$^{8}/_{160}$	5%	$^{12}/_{143}$	8%	NS
Dura torn	$^{21}/_{133}$	16%	$^{52}/_{175}$	30%	<0.01
Frontal	$^{13}/_{123}$	11%	$^{36}/_{154}$	23%	<0.01
Temporo-parietal	$^{14}/_{180}$	8%	$^{30}/_{162}$	19%	<0.01
Occipital	$^{0}/_{31}$	0%	$^{2}/_{18}$	11%	<0.05

Other Non-focal Features Affecting Incidence of Late Epilepsy

The single factor which most significantly and most consistently increased the incidence of late epilepsy was *prolonged PTA*. As might be expected this was often associated with other factors which in themselves have a high risk of late epilepsy, namely focal signs, dural tearing and age over 16 years (16/17). But in fact epilepsy was more frequent when PTA was prolonged in these subgroups as in all others (16/18). When depressed fractures as a whole are considered (regardless of any other feature of injury) it transpires that only when PTA exceeds 24 hours is the late epilepsy rate significantly greater after depressed fracture, as compared with other injuries (16/19). That is not to say that under certain circumstances depressed fracture with a shorter PTA may not be associated with a higher late epilepsy rate than obtains for injuries without depressed fracture (16/20).

16/17 *Association of various features with duration of PTA*

Feature	Frequency of feature in cases with		P
	PTA $<$ 24 hours	PTA $>$ 24 hours	
$>$ 16 years	$321/698$ 46%	$158/230$ 69%	<0.001
Focal signs	$98/698$ 14%	$91/230$ 40%	<0.001
Dura torn (compound)	$269/616$ 44%	$145/209$ 69%	<0.001

16/18 *Influence of PTA on the incidence of late epilepsy after depressed fracture with different features*

	PTA $<$ 24 hours	PTA $>$ 24 hours	P
$<$ 16 years	$14/286$ 5%	$15/54$ 28%	<0.001
$>$ 16 years	$32/234$ 14%	$38/112$ 34%	<0.001
No early epilepsy	$37/462$ 8%	$40/143$ 28%	<0.001
After early epilepsy	$8/58$ 14%	$13/23$ 57%	<0.001
No focal signs	$34/444$ 8%	$26/94$ 28%	<0.001
With focal signs	$12/76$ 16%	$27/72$ 38%	<0.01
Closed	$3/65$ 5%	$4/16$ 25%	<0.01
Compound	$42/454$ 9%	$49/150$ 33%	<0.001
Dura intact	$8/249$ 3%	$12/50$ 24%	<0.001
Dura torn	$34/206$ 17%	$37/100$ 37%	<0.001

16/19 *Effect of depressed fracture and PTA on incidence of late epilepsy*

	PTA $<$ 24 hours	PTA $>$ 24 hours	P
No depressed fracture	$8/125$ 6%	$9/98$ 9%	NS
Depressed fracture	$45/520$ 9%	$53/166$ 32%	<0.001
P	NS	<0.001	

16/20 *Features which significantly increase late epilepsy incidence in depressed fracture with < 24 hours PTA, compared with other injuries*

No depressed fracture	$^{27}/_{832}$	3%

Depressed fracture with < 24 hours PTA			P v no depressed fracture
> 16 years	$^{32}/_{234}$	14%	< 0.001
Compound	$^{42}/_{454}$	9%	< 0.001
Compound, dura torn	$^{34}/_{206}$	17%	< 0.001
With focal signs	$^{12}/_{76}$	16%	< 0.001
After early epilepsy	$^{8}/_{58}$	14%	< 0.001

Early epilepsy also increased the incidence of late epilepsy after depressed fracture, but not significantly so; and depressed fracture did not add to the already high risk of epilepsy when an early fit had already occurred (16/21). It is the opposite interaction to that associated with PTA (16/19). Early epilepsy did not show an association with other features which lead to late epilepsy (16/22), and in predisposing to late epilepsy the influence of early epilepsy was neither as marked or as consistent as was that of prolonged PTA (compare 16/18 with 16/23).

16/21 *Effect of depressed fracture and early epilepsy on incidence of late epilepsy*

	No early epilepsy		Early epilepsy		P
No depressed fracture	$^{11}/_{196}$	6%	$^{21}/_{91}$	23%	< 0.001
Depressed fracture	$^{63}/_{396}$	16%	$^{13}/_{51}$	26%	NS
P	< 0.001		NS		

16/22 *Association of various features with early epilepsy*

| Feature | Frequency of feature in cases with | | P |
	No early epilepsy	Early epilepsy	
< 16 years	$^{441}/_{851}$ 52%	$^{47}/_{96}$ 49%	NS
PTA > 24 hours	$^{203}/_{831}$ 24%	$^{27}/_{96}$ 28%	NS
Focal signs	$^{167}/_{851}$ 20%	$^{25}/_{96}$ 26%	NS
Compound fracture	$^{758}/_{851}$ 89%	$^{82}/_{96}$ 85%	NS
Dura torn	$^{372}/_{758}$ 49%	$^{47}/_{82}$ 57%	NS

16/23 *Influence of early epilepsy on incidence of late epilepsy after depressed fractures with different features*

	No early epilepsy	After early epilepsy	P
PTA < 24 hours	$^{37}/_{462}$ 8%	$^{8}/_{58}$ 14%	NS
PTA > 24 hours	$^{40}/_{143}$ 28%	$^{13}/_{23}$ 57%	< 0.01
No focal signs	$^{48}/_{487}$ 10%	$^{14}/_{59}$ 24%	< 0.01
After focal signs	$^{33}/_{126}$ 25%	$^{7}/_{22}$ 32%	NS
Dura intact	$^{17}/_{273}$ 6%	$^{3}/_{30}$ 10%	NS
Dura torn	$^{57}/_{266}$ 21%	$^{16}/_{43}$ 37%	NS

Focal Features

1. Site of Fracture

The detailed analysis of the non-missile series results in figures in several areas which are too small for reliable statistics, but it serves to indicate that there is no one area with a strikingly different incidence of epilepsy, early or late (16/24). When the epilepsy incidence for various larger areas is analysed, the only significant difference is the lower rate for occipital

16/24 *Epilepsy after non-missile injuries* (Detailed series, see Fig. 9)

	Early		Late	
1. Fronto-polar — high sagittal	$^0/_3$	0%	$^0/_2$	50%
2. Fronto-polar — low sagittal	$^4/_{17}$	24%	$^5/_{15}$	33%
3. Fronto-polar — upper lateral	$^4/_{27}$	15%	$^5/_{20}$	25%
4. Fronto-polar — low lateral	$^6/_{41}$	15%	$^3/_{25}$	12%
5. Upper lateral frontal	$^4/_{22}$	18%	$^4/_{20}$	20%
6. Lower lateral frontal	$^0/_8$	0%	$^1/_6$	17%
7. Upper anterior parietal	$^5/_{43}$	12%	$^6/_{31}$	19%
8. Lower anterior parietal	$^2/_{18}$	11%	$^2/_{17}$	12%
9. Upper posterior parietal	$^4/_{70}$	6%	$^3/_{47}$	6%
10. Low posterior parietal	$^3/_{27}$	11%	$^2/_{17}$	12%
11. Temporal	$^0/_6$	(0%)	$^1/_5$	(20%)
12. Occipital	$^2/_{18}$	11%	$^0/_{13}$	0%

16/25 *Epilepsy at different sites by bones of skull*

Detailed series	Early epilepsy		Late epilepsy	
Frontal bone	$^{18}/_{118}$	15%	$^{18}/_{88}$	21%
Parietal bone	$^{14}/_{158}$	9%	$^{14}/_{112}$	13%
Temporal bone	$^0/_6$	(0%)	$^1/_5$	(20%)
Occipital bone	$^2/_{18}$	11%	$^0/_{13}$	0%
Frontal	$^{18}/_{118}$	15%	$^{18}/_{88}$	21%
Temporo-parietal	$^{14}/_{164}$	9%	$^{15}/_{117}$	13%
P	NS		NS	
Total series				
Frontal	$^{41}/_{386}$	11%	$^{48}/_{277}$	17%
Temporo-parietal	$^{49}/_{453}$	11%	$^{44}/_{342}$	13%
Occipital	$^3/_{72}$	4%	$^2/_{49}$	4%
P (occipital vs. rest)	NS		<0.05	

16/26   *Epilepsy at different sites by lobes of brain*

	Missile Russell and Whitty		Non-missile			
			Early		*Late*	
A Pre-frontal and inferior frontal	$^{63}/_{160}$	39%	$^{14}/_{88}$	16%	$^{13}/_{62}$	21%
B Motor and pre-motor	$^{70}/_{127}$	55%	$^{11}/_{92}$	12%	$^{13}/_{74}$	18%
C Parietal lobe	$^{111}/_{170}$	65%	$^{6}/_{67}$	9%	$^{3}/_{51}$	6%
D Temporal lobe	$^{27}/_{71}$	38%	$^{0}/_{6}$	(0%)	$^{1}/_{5}$	(20%)
E Occipital lobe	$^{28}/_{73}$	38%	$^{3}/_{47}$	6%	$^{2}/_{26}$	8%
B + C (Central zone)	$^{181}/_{297}$	61%	$^{17}/_{159}$	11%	$^{16}/_{125}$	13%
A + D + E	$^{118}/_{304}$	39%	$^{17}/_{141}$	12%	$^{16}/_{93}$	17%
P	< 0.001		NS		NS	
A + B (Frontal lobe)	$^{133}/_{287}$	46%	$^{25}/_{180}$	14%	$^{26}/_{136}$	19%
C + D + E	$^{166}/_{314}$	53%	$^{9}/_{120}$	8%	$^{6}/_{82}$	7%
P	NS		NS		< 0.02	

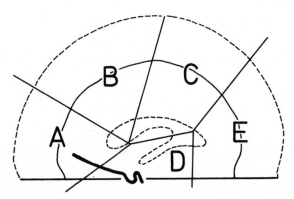

Fig. 11. Lobes of brain (*after Russell 1947*).

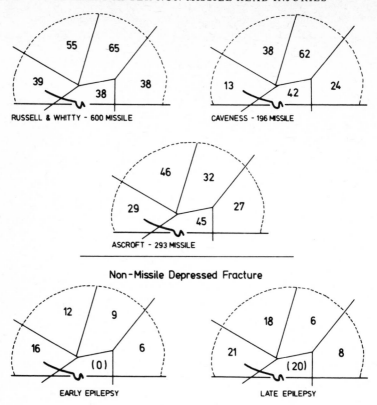

Fig. 12. Incidence of epilepsy by lobe involved; early and late are identified only for non-missile series.

fracture (16/25). Fractures of the temporal *bone* are so unusual that the epilepsy rate cannot be reliably calculated; as a result of the rarity of temporal fractures the figures for temporo-parietal fractures in the total series in fact refer largely to parietal bone fractures.

If this detailed series of non-missile fractures is now analysed by *lobes* it is possible to make comparisons with the incidence of epilepsy after missile injuries (published series of which do not distinguish between early and late epilepsy). Russell and Whitty found that fracture adjacent to the central sulcus (his areas B and C, Fig. 11) had a significantly higher epilepsy incidence, but this was less obvious in the other missile series and

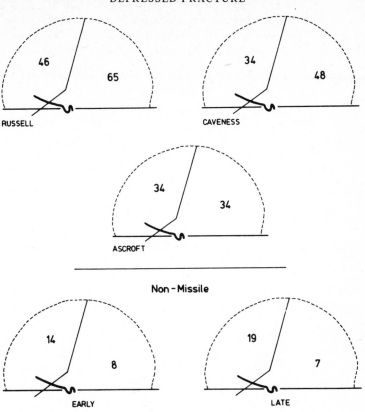

Fig. 13. Incidence of epilepsy on either side of Rolandic Sulcus.

not evident in the non-missile series (16/26). For the non-missile series, when analysed by lobes, frontal lobe fractures prove to be more often followed by epilepsy, both early and late, but this difference was significant only for late epilepsy (Fig. 12, 13).

2. Focal Signs

The development of any signs of dysfunction of the cerebral hemisphere, even if only temporary, significantly increases the incidence of late epilepsy (16/27). The risk is greater if the symptoms persist more than 6 months, but not significantly so (16/28). Signs included are any degree of motor or sensory hemiparesis, including hemianopia, or dysphasia. As might be expected patients with focal signs included an undue proportion with prolonged PTA and with dural tearing (16/29), but this did not wholly account for the increased incidence of epilepsy associated with focal signs, because this was observed after several different types of injury (16/30).

3. Compounding

It might be expected that late epilepsy would be commoner after compound fracture than closed, which indeed was the case although the difference is not significant (16/31). Other features of injury are similar in closed and compound fractures (16/32); compound fractures did not carry a significantly increased epilepsy risk in any of the subgroups (16/33). This rather surprising finding may be explained by some selection of the closed fractures which are referred to neurosurgical units. Considering that even compound fractures are not infrequently overlooked it seems probable that a number of closed fractures go undetected altogether. Even when recognised there is not as definite an indication for operation as with compound fractures, and it is likely that those referred for specialist opinion included more with early epilepsy, with focal signs and with prolonged PTA than would be found in a completely unselected series (if such a series could ever be collected).

4. Dural tearing

Students of traumatic epilepsy have always emphasised the importance of dural tearing (or penetration) as a factor contributing to an increased risk of late epilepsy; this is usually attributed to the more extensive brain damage liable to occur when the dura is breached, and also the possibility of infection. The present study certainly confirms these views, in that late epilepsy was much more frequent when the dura was torn (16/34), and both prolonged PTA and focal signs were significantly more common after

16/27   *Signs and incidence of late epilepsy*

No signs	$^{47}/_{511}$	9%
Signs of cerebral hemisphere dysfunction	$^{53}/_{182}$	29%
P		< 0.001

16/28   *Effect of duration of signs on incidence of late epilepsy after depressed fracture*

Signs resolved within six months	$^{24}/_{101}$	24%
Signs persisting for > six months	$^{29}/_{81}$	36%
P		NS

16/29   *Features in cases with and without focal signs*

	Frequency of feature in cases with			
Feature	No focal signs		Focal signs	P
< 16 years	$^{365}/_{756}$	48%	$^{124}/_{192}$ 65%	< 0.001
PTA > 24 hours	$^{139}/_{739}$	19%	$^{91}/_{189}$ 48%	< 0.001
Dura torn	$^{294}/_{663}$	44%	$^{126}/_{178}$ 71%	< 0.001
Early epilepsy	$^{71}/_{756}$	9%	$^{25}/_{192}$ 13%	NS

compound fractures when there was dural tearing (16/35). Under a wide range of circumstances dural tearing increased the late epilepsy rate, although this did not reach significance for injuries with prolonged PTA, which without dural tearing already have a high risk of late epilepsy (16/36).

16/30   *Influence of focal signs on incidence of late epilepsy after depressed fracture*

	No focal signs		With focal signs		P
PTA < 24 hours	$34/444$	8%	$12/76$	16%	< 0.05
PTA > 24 hours	$26/94$	28%	$27/72$	33%	NS
No early epilepsy	$48/487$	10%	$32/126$	25%	< 0.001
After early epilepsy	$14/59$	24%	$7/22$	32%	NS
Dura intact	$17/263$	6%	$3/40$	8%	NS
Dura torn	$41/212$	19%	$33/97$	34%	< 0.001

16/31   *Incidence of late epilepsy after closed and compound depressed fracture*

Closed	$7/82$	9%
Compound	$93/611$	15%
P	NS	

16/32   *Association of various features with compound depressed fracture*

	Frequency of feature in cases which are			
Feature	Closed		Compound	P
> 16 years	$41/107$	38%	$448/840$	53%	< 0.001
PTA > 24 hours	$21/103$	20%	$209/825$	25%	NS
Early epilepsy	$14/107$	13%	$82/840$	10%	NS
Focal signs	$14/107$	13%	$178/840$	21%	NS

16/33   *Influence of compound depressed fracture on incidence of late epilepsy with various features*

Feature	Closed		Compound		P
< 16 years	$^2/_{52}$	4%	$^{29}/_{293}$	10%	NS
> 16 years	$^5/_{30}$	17%	$^{65}/_{319}$	20%	NS
PTA < 24 hours	$^3/_{65}$	5%	$^{42}/_{454}$	9%	NS
PTA > 24 hours	$^4/_{16}$	25%	$^{49}/_{150}$	33%	NS
No early epilepsy	$^5/_{74}$	8%	$^{74}/_{539}$	14%	NS
After early epilepsy	$^2/_8$	25%	$^{19}/_{73}$	26%	NS
No focal signs	$^4/_{71}$	6%	$^{58}/_{475}$	12%	NS
Focal signs	$^3/_{11}$	27%	$^{36}/_{137}$	26%	NS

16/34   *Incidence of late epilepsy after compound depressed fracture*

Dura intact	$^{20}/_{303}$	7%
Dura torn	$^{73}/_{309}$	24%
P		< 0.001

16/35   *Association of various features with dural tearing*

Feature	Frequency of feature in cases with				P
	Dura intact		Dura torn		
< 16 years	$^{204}/_{420}$	49%	$^{244}/_{420}$	58%	< 0.01
PTA > 24 hours	$^{64}/_{411}$	16%	$^{145}/_{413}$	35%	< 0.001
Focal signs	$^{52}/_{420}$	12%	$^{126}/_{420}$	30%	< 0.001
Early epilepsy	$^{35}/_{420}$	8%	$^{47}/_{420}$	11%	NS

16/36   *Influence of dural tearing on incidence of late epilepsy after compound depressed fracture*

	Dura intact		Dura torn		P
PTA $<$ 24 hours	$^8/_{249}$	3%	$^{34}/_{206}$	17%	<0.001
PTA $>$ 24 hours	$^{12}/_{50}$	24%	$^{37}/_{100}$	37%	NS
No focal signs	$^{17}/_{263}$	7%	$^{41}/_{212}$	19%	<0.001
With focal signs	$^3/_{40}$	8%	$^{33}/_{97}$	34%	<0.001
No early epilepsy	$^{17}/_{273}$	6%	$^{57}/_{266}$	21%	<0.001
After early epilepsy	$^3/_{30}$	10%	$^{16}/_{43}$	37%	<0.01

5. Elevation of the Fracture

It remains to consider whether different forms of treatment have any influence on the incidence of late epilepsy. The prediction that traumatic epilepsy might largely disappear once elevation became routine was obviously over-optimistic, but it seems worthwhile considering whether elevation in fact reduces the risk. Operation for compound fracture is primarily carried out to minimise the risk of infection but it is not unusual to hear advanced, as one reason for operating on closed fractures, the belief (or hope) that the chance of late epilepsy will be reduced. It is not easy to find a series of unelevated fractures which is well-matched with a series of elevated fractures, because those which are left unoperated are likely to be less serious or complicated. Closed fractures, however, are quite commonly left untreated and in practice quite a number of compound fractures are dealt with by simple debridement only. The usual reason for this is proximity of the fracture to one of the intracranial venous sinuses, such that elevation would carry the risk of serious haemorrhage. But some fractures are not elevated because the patient is referred to a neurosurgeon only after adequate scalp suturing has been completed elsewhere; this may have resulted from failure to appreciate that a depressed fracture lay underneath, or there may have been a deliberate decision to suture the scalp prior to long-distance transfer to a neurosurgical unit. Whether secondary, delayed debridement is undertaken under these circumstances depends largely on how efficient the scalp toilet and suturing appears to have been. Also whether there has been delay of a day or two so that the wound is already almost healed.

16/37 *Incidence of late epilepsy after depressed fractures differently treated*

	Closed		Compound	
No elevation	$3/34$	9%	$5/87$	6%
Elevation	$3/47$	6%	$89/524$	17%
P	NS		<0.01	

In any event it proved possible to collect a series of fractures which had not been elevated; and for the closed fractures there was no difference in the late epilepsy incidence, when compared with elevated fractures (16/37). Unelevated compound fractures had a similar epilepsy rate to that for closed fractures; but elevated compound fractures had a higher incidence of epilepsy, no doubt because these included all the dural penetrating injuries. However, prolonged PTA and focal signs were equally frequent in the elevated and unelevated fractures.

6. Bone Removed or Replaced

After formal elevation has been undertaken the bone fragments may be discarded or replaced. All writings about missile wounds emphasise the importance of the removing all fragments, which after such injuries are often grossly contaminated and usually fractured into many tiny pieces; subsequently a cranioplasty may be required. In the treatment of civilian depressed fractures there have been claims from time to time that replacement of large fragments as a mosaic is safe under certain circumstances. Kriss and his colleagues (1969) showed that infection was no more common after such a procedure and this has been confirmed in Glasgow (Jennett and Miller, 1972), and in Rotterdam (Braakman, 1972) the method having been widely employed in both these cities.

Epilepsy was rather more frequent when the bone fragments had been removed but without a cranioplasty being performed (either at once or subsequently) (16/38). It might be suspected that bone was more likely to be removed after more severe injuries, but prolonged PTA was no more common in such cases except in the cranioplasty group (16/39). When comparison is made separately for those with PTA greater and less than 24 hours there proves to be no significant difference in the epilepsy rate whether the bone is replaced or removed, but it is higher in those cases in which cranioplasty was necessary (16/40). Whether cranioplasty itself

16/38   *Incidence of late epilepsy after compound depressed fracture differently treated*

Bone fragments replaced	$^{23}/_{251}$	9%	
Bone fragments removed — no cranioplasty	$^{23}/_{136}$	17%	$P < 0.05$
Bone fragments removed — cranioplasty	$^{26}/_{68}$	38%	$P < 0.001$

Relationships: $P < 0.001$ overall.

16/39   *Frequency of PTA > 24 hours in fractures differently treated*

Bone replaced	$^{52}/_{247}$	21%	
Bone removed — no cranioplasty	$^{33}/_{136}$	24%	P NS
Cranioplasty	$^{24}/_{220}$	36%	P NS

Overall $P < 0.01$.

16/40   *Interaction of bone treatment and PTA on incidence of late epilepsy*

	PTA < 24 hours		PTA > 24 hours	
Bone replaced	$^{11}/_{195}$ 6%		$^{12}/_{52}$ 23%	
Bone removed — no cranioplasty	$^{12}/_{103}$ 12%	P NS	$^{11}/_{33}$ 33%	P NS
Bone removed — cranioplasty	$^{11}/_{42}$ 26%	$P < 0.05$	$^{13}/_{24}$ 54%	P NS

contributes to the higher epilepsy rate is uncertain; it seems more likely that cranioplasty was more readily resorted to after more severe and complicated injuries, and it is even possible that one reason for a cranioplasty might sometimes be the development of epilepsy, but from the data available no conclusion could be reached about this. It does seem certain, however, that the risk of epilepsy is no reason for removing bone fragments, nor if they have been removed is it a good reason for recommending cranioplasty.

This association between high epilepsy rate and cranioplasty has been commented on by Walker and Erculei (1963) in relation to missile injuries. They attribute it to the greater tendency for cranioplasty to be done after more severe wounds. They could find no evidence that cranioplasty had any real effect on post-traumatic epilepsy.

7. Infection

This was noted in 8% of 948 depressed fractures, and early epilepsy was somewhat more frequent (15%) with infected fractures (10%). Late epilepsy however, occurred significantly more often after infected fractures (16/41).

The relation between epilepsy and infection after missile wounds is conflicting. Certainly there has been no obvious reduction in the epilepsy rate concomitant with the dramatic lowering of the occurrence of infection in successive wars (15/1, 2, page 90). Likewise in dural penetrating injuries Russell found no difference in the epilepsy rate whether or not there had been infection, but others have reported a higher incidence of epilepsy after infection (16/42).

16/41 *Effect of infection on incidence of late epilepsy*

Infection	$16/51$	31%
No infection	$85/643$	13%
P		<0.001

Interaction Between Features

Preceding analyses have identified four features which are associated with an increased risk of late epilepsy after depressed fracture — prolonged PTA, focal signs, dural tearing and the occurrence of early epilepsy. These features are not independent variables, but the dependence between them is complex; as a result the extent to which, when more than one feature occurs in the same patient, there is an additive epileptogenic effect is also variable.

When the interaction between **pairs of these features** is explored, in respect of the incidence of late epilepsy, a number of different patterns is discovered.

16/42 *Interaction of PTA and early epilepsy on incidence of late epilepsy after depressed fracture*

	PTA < 24 hours	PTA > 24 hours	P
No early epilepsy	$^{37}/_{462}$ 8%	$^{40}/_{143}$ 28%	< 0.001
After early epilepsy	$^{8}/_{58}$ 14%	$^{13}/_{23}$ 57%	< 0.001
P	NS	< 0.01	

(a) Both features are additive, which is to say that when both occurred together the incidence of late epilepsy was significantly greater than with either alone. This relationship held for early epilepsy and PTA (16/42), and for focal signs and dural tearing (16/43). In each of these sets the opposite effect was also observed, that when one feature was absent (prolonged PTA in 16/42, or dural tearing 16/43) the other feature did not increase the epilepsy incidence. From this data it can be concluded that long PTA is a more potent epileptogenic feature than is early epilepsy, and dural tearing than focal signs, because each of these features increased the epilepsy rate regardless of the other.

(b) Three other pairs of features show a higher epilepsy rate when both features occur together, but this was not significantly greater than one of the other combinations (of one feature present and the other absent). Thus, focal signs in 16/44, and dural tearing in 16/45, did not significantly increase the epilepsy rate when PTA was prolonged; in 16/46 early epilepsy did not significantly increase the epilepsy rate when the dura was torn.

16/43 *Interaction of focal signs and dural tearing on incidence of late epilepsy*

	Dura intact	Dura torn	P
No focal signs	$^{17}/_{263}$ 6%	$^{41}/_{212}$ 19%	< 0.001
Focal signs	$^{3}/_{40}$ 8%	$^{33}/_{97}$ 34%	< 0.001
P	NS	< 0.01	

16/44 *Interaction of focal signs and PTA on incidence of late epilepsy*

	PTA < 24 hours		PTA > 24 hours		P
No focal signs	$^{34}/_{444}$	8%	$^{26}/_{94}$	28%	< 0.001
Focal signs	$^{12}/_{76}$	16%	$^{27}/_{72}$	33%	< 0.01
P	< 0.05		NS		

16/45 *Interaction of dural state and PTA on incidence of late epilepsy*

	PTA < 24 hours		PTA > 24 hours		P
Dura intact	$^{8}/_{249}$	3%	$^{12}/_{50}$	24%	< 0.001
Dura torn	$^{34}/_{205}$	17%	$^{37}/_{100}$	37%	< 0.001
P	< 0.001		NS		

16/46 *Interaction of dural state and early epilepsy on incidence of late epilepsy*

	Dura intact		Dura torn		P
No early epilepsy	$^{17}/_{273}$	6%	$^{57}/_{266}$	21%	< 0.001
After early epilepsy	$^{3}/_{30}$	10%	$^{16}/_{43}$	37%	< 0.01
P	NS		NS		

16/47   *Interaction of focal signs and early epilepsy on incidence of late epilepsy after depressed fracture*

	No early epilepsy	After early epilepsy	P
No focal signs	$^{48}/_{487}$ 10%	$^{14}/_{59}$ 24%	< 0.01
Focal signs	$^{32}/_{126}$ 25%	$^{7}/_{22}$ 32%	NS
P	< 0.001	NS	

(c) With one pair of features only the combination did not give a significantly higher incidence of epilepsy than did either of the features alone (16/47).

Combinations of more than two factors. In general a more accurate estimate can be made about the risk of epilepsy if three factors are known rather than two. But because some factors are dominant to others there are some combinations of two factors which are as powerful predictors as other combinations of three, or even four, factors. When epilepsy rates are set out in rank order, when two factors only are known, it is evident that the rate is always higher when two factors are positive than when only one is; one factor positive gives a higher rate than when two factors are negative, with a single exception (16/48).

The dominant influence of PTA is again evident from this analysis. When the PTA is unknown the range of risk of late epilepsy, given only two factors known, is from 6-37% (16/49a); three risk levels can be identified, according to the other factors (16/49b). When PTA is known the range of incidence expands to 3-60% (16/50a). Different levels of risk can then be identified according to whether PTA is greater than 24 hours (16/50b), or is less prolonged (16/50c).

When the effect of adding a third factor is explored, problems arise in some sub-groups because the samples are so small. In 16/51-54 the effect of an additional factor is set out, each table dealing with the addition of a different factor. In many instances a wide difference appeared between the two sub-groups which resulted from adding a third factor, but in only 13 of 44 instances (30%) was this difference statistically significant (insignificance usually being due to the smallness of the sub-groups). A significant difference was more often achieved when the additional factor was duration of PTA, which is yet further evidence of

16/48 *Incidence of late epilepsy after compound depressed fracture. Two factors known*

PTA > 24 hours	Dura torn	Focal signs	Early epilepsy	% Late epilepsy	
+	□	□	+	60	two factors +ve
+	+	□	□	37	
□	+	□	+	37	
□	+	+	□	34	
+	□	+	□	33	
□	□	+	+	32	
+	□	□	○	28	one factor +ve
+	□	○	□	28	
□	□	+	○	25	
+	○	□	□	24	
□	□	○	+	24	
□	+	□	○	21	
□	+	○	□	19	
○	+	□	□	17	
○	□	+	□	16	
○	□	□	+	13	
□	□	○	○	10	○ factor +ve (except focal signs)
○	□	□	○	9	
□	○	+	□	8	
○	□	○	□	8	
□	○	○	□	6	
○	○	□	□	3	

(Arranged in rank order of epilepsy incidence)

+ = positive;   ○ = negative;   □ = no information.

the importance of this particular item of data (16/55). However, when the influence of each factor alone is considered, given varying combinations of the other two factors, varying ranges of risk are found (16/56). At the two ends of this scale it is possible to indicate that if the dura is torn then the risk of epilepsy is always over 20%, whatever the other factors; and if the PTA is less than 24 hours than the risk of epilepsy is always less than 22%, whatever the other factors.

Incidence of late epilepsy after depressed fracture
16/49a   *Two factors–PTA not known*

Dural tearing	Focal signs	Early epilepsy	Late epilepsy
+	□	+	37%
+	+	□	34%
□	+	+	32%
□	+	○	25%
□	○	+	24%
+	□	○	21%
+	○	□	19%
□	○	○	10%
○	+	□	8%
○	○	□	6%
			Range = 6-37%

+ = positive;   ○ = negative;   □ = no information.

16/49b   *Two factors–PTA unknown*

6–10%	19–25%	33–37%
No factors positive (except focal signs)	Any *one* factor positive (except focal signs)	Any *two* factors of: early epilepsy dura torn focal signs

Incidence of late epilepsy after depressed fracture.
16/50a   *Two factors—PTA known*

PTA > 24 hours	Dural tear	Focal signs	Early epilepsy	%
+	□	□	+	60
+	+	□	□	37
+	□	+	□	33
+	□	□	○	28
+	□	○	□	28
+	○	□	□	24
○	+	□	□	17
○	□	+	□	16
○	□	□	+	13
○	□	□	○	9
○	□	○	□	8
○	○	□	□	3
			Range =	3–60%

(Arranged in rank order of epilepsy incidence)

+ = positive;   ○ = negative;   □ = no information.

16/50b   *PTA >24 hours given one other feature*

24–28%	33–37%	60%
Neither dural tear nor early epilepsy nor focal signs	Dura torn or Focal signs	After early epilepsy

16/50c   *Incidence of late epilepsy after depressed fracture with PTA <24 hours given one other feature*

3–5%	5–10%	14–17%
< 16 years or Closed or Dura intact	Neither dural tear nor early epilepsy nor focal signs	> 16 years or After early epilepsy or Focal signs or Dura torn

16/51   *The effect of 3rd factor on incidence of late epilepsy after compound depressed fracture (additional factor PTA)*

Two factors	I_2	Three factors		I_3	P
1 2 3 4		1 2 3 4			
□ + ○ □	19%	○ + ○ □	$25/161$	15%	NS
		+ + ○ □	$14/48$	29%	
□ ○ ○ □	6%	○ ○ ○ □	$7/225$	3%	< 0.001
		+ ○ ○ □	$10/34$	29%	
□ + □ ○	21%	○ + □ ○	$28/179$	16%	< 0.01
		+ + □ ○	$27/84$	32%	
□ + + □	34%	○ + + □	$10/45$	22%	NS
		+ + + □	$23/59$	39%	
□ □ + +		○ □ + +	$1/11$	9%	< 0.02
		+ □ + +	$6/10$	60%	
□ □ + ○	25%	○ □ + ○	$10/58$	17%	NS
		+ □ + ○	$19/58$	33%	
□ + □ +	37%	+ + □ +	$10/16$	63%	< 0.01
		○ + □ +	$6/27$	22%	
□ □ ○ ○	10%	○ □ ○ ○	$26/344$	8%	< 0.001
		+ □ ○ ○	$18/72$	25%	
□ □ ○ +	24%	+ □ ○ +	$6/10$	60%	< 0.01
		○ □ ○ +	$6/42$	14%	
□ ○ + □	8%	○ ○ + □	$1/24$	4%	NS
		+ ○ + □	$2/16$	13%	
Range 8–37%;				Range 3–63%.	

Factors, reading from left to right, 1 = PTA > 24 hours, 2 = dura torn, 3 = focal signs, 4 = early epilepsy.

+ = positive;   ○ = negative;   □ = no information.

Incidence of epilepsy (%) based on 2 factors (I_2) and on 3 factors (I_3).

16/52 *The effect of 3rd factor on incidence of late epilepsy after compound depressed fracture (additional factor **dural state**)*

Two factors 1 2 3 4	I_2	Three factors 1 2 3 4		I_3	P
+ □ □ +	60%	+ ○ □ +	2/4	50%	NS
		+ + □ +	10/16	63%	
○ □ + □	16%	○ ○ + □	1/24	4%	NS
		○ + + □	10/45	22%	
+ □ ○ □	28%	+ + ○ □	14/48	29%	NS
		+ ○ ○ □	10/34	29%	
□ □ + ○	25%	□ ○ + ○	2/27	5%	< 0.001
		□ + + ○	27/79	34%	
+ + □ □	37%	+ + + □	23/59	39%	NS
		+ + ○ □	14/48	29%	
+ □ □ ○	28%	+ + □ ○	27/84	32%	NS
		+ ○ □ ○	10/46	22%	
○ □ □ +	13%	○ ○ □ +	1/26	4%	NS
		○ + □ +	6/27	22%	
□ □ ○ +	24%	□ ○ ○ +	2/27	7%	NS
		□ + ○ +	10/45	20%	
□ □ + +		□ ○ + +	1/3	33%	NS
		□ + + +	6/18	33%	
+ □ + □	33%	+ ○ + □	2/16	13%	NS
		+ + + □	23/59	39%	
○ □ ○ □	8%	○ ○ ○ □	7/225	3%	< 0.001
		○ + ○ □	25/161	16%	
□ □ ○ ○	10%	□ ○ ○ ○	15/236	6%	< 0.001
		□ + ○ ○	31/187	17%	
○ □ □ ○	9%	○ + □ ○	28/179	16%	< 0.001
		○ ○ □ ○	7/223	3%	
Range 8–60%		Range 3–63%.			

Factors, reading from left to right, 1 = PTA > 24 hours, 2 = dura torn, 3 = focal signs, 4 = early epilepsy.

+ = positive;   ○ = negative;   □ = no information.

Incidence of epilepsy (%) based on 2 factors (I_2) and on 3 factors (I_3).

16/53 *The effect of 3rd factor on incidence of late epilepsy after compound depressed fracture (additional factor focal signs)*

Two factors	I_2	Three factors		I_3	P
1 2 3 4		1 2 3 4			
+ □ □ O	28%	+ □ O O	$18/72$	25%	NS
		+ □ + O	$19/58$	33%	
O + □ □	17%	O + □ O	$28/179$	16%	NS
		O + □ +	$6/27$	22%	
+ O □ □	24%	+ O O □	$10/34$	29%	NS
		+ O + □	$2/16$	13%	
O O □ □	3%	O O O □	$7/225$	3%	NS
		O O + □	$1/24$	4%	
O □ □ +	13%	O □ O +	$6/42$	14%	NS
		O □ + +	$1/11$	9%	
O □ □ O	9%	O □ O O	$26/344$	8%	< 0.02
		O □ + O	$10/58$	17%	
+ □ □ +	60%	+ □ O +	$6/10$	60%	NS
		+ □ + +	$6/10$	60%	
□ + □ +	37%	□ + O +	$10/25$	40%	NS
		□ + + +	$6/18$	33%	
□ + □ O	21%	□ + O O	$31/187$	17%	< 0.01
		□ + + O	$27/79$	34%	
Range 3–60%		Range 3–60%			

Factors, reading from left to right, 1 = PTA > 24 hours, 2 = dura torn, 3 = focal signs, 4 = early epilepsy.

+ = positive; O = negative; □ = no information.

Incidence of epilepsy (%) based on 2 factors (I_2) and on 3 factors (I_3).

16/54 *The effect of 3rd factor on incidence of late epilepsy after compound depressed fracture (additional factor **early epilepsy**)*

Two factors 1 2 3 4	I_2	Three factors 1 2 3 4		I_3	P
□ + ○ □	19%	□ + ○ +	10/25	40%	} < 0.01
		□ + ○ ○	31/187	17%	
+ □ ○ □	28%	+ □ ○ ○	18/72	25%	} NS
		+ □ ○ +	6/10	60%	
+ ○ □ □	24%	+ ○ □ ○	10/45	22%	} NS
		+ ○ □ +	2/4	50%	
□ ○ ○ □	6%	□ ○ ○ +	2/27	7%	} NS
		□ ○ ○ ○	15/236	6%	
+ + □ □	37%	+ + □ ○	27/84	32%	} NS
		+ + □ +	10/16	63%	
○ □ + □	16%	○ □ + ○	10/58	17%	} NS
		○ □ + +	1/11	9%	
□ ○ + □	8%	□ ○ + ○	2/37	5%	} NS
		□ ○ + +	1/3	33%	
○ □ ○ □	8%	○ □ ○ +	6/42	14%	} NS
		○ □ ○ ○	26/344	8%	
○ + □ □	17%	○ + ○ □	25/161	16%	} NS
		○ + + □	10/45	22%	
+ □ + □	33%	+ □ + ○	19/58	33%	} NS
		+ □ + +	6/10	60%	
□ + + □	34%	□ + + ○	27/79	34%	} NS
		□ + + +	6/18	33%	
○ ○ □ □	3%	○ ○ □ ○	7/223	3%	} NS
		○ ○ □ +	1/26	4%	
Range 3–37%;		Range 3–63%.			

Factors, reading from left to right, 1 = PTA > 24 hours, 2 = dura torn, 3 = focal signs, 4 = early epilepsy.

+ = positive;   ○ = negative;   □ = no information.

Incidence of epilepsy (%) based on 2 factors (I_2) and on 3 factors (I_3).

16/55   *Frequency of significant difference appearing by addition of different third factors*

Added factor (either positive or negative)	Number of subgroups significantly distinguished	
PTA	$^6/_{10}$	60%
Dural state	$^4/_{13}$	31%
Focal signs	$^2/_9$	22%
Early epilepsy	$^1/_{12}$	8%

16/56   *Range of epilepsy risks associated with each factor, according to different pairs of other factors*

Dural tear	21–63%	(always $\geqslant 21\%$)
PTA $>$ 24 hours	13–63%	
Early epilepsy	4–63%	
Focal signs	4–60%	
No focal signs	3–60%	
Dura intact	3–50%	
No early epilepsy	3–34%	
PTA $<$ 24 hours	3–22%	(always $\leqslant 22\%$)

When the influence of a fourth factor is considered the numbers become so small that useful conclusions can be drawn about only one sub-group — those without early epilepsy. The range of incidence in such cases is not increased by adding a fourth factor, but a significant difference is found in 5 out of 24 sub-groups derived from this addition (21%). The number of groups which became significantly different was similar whether additional information was about duration of PTA or the state of the dura, but adding focal signs led to much less differentiation. Thus we can conclude that if data is available about the PTA or dural state then almost as accurate a prediction can be made as when there is also information about focal signs or early epilepsy. But in the absence of

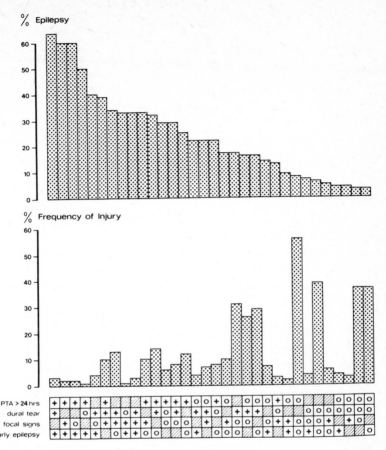

Fig. 14. The frequency with which different combinations of factors occurred is displayed below the incidence of late epilepsy associated with each combination (three factors of four available).

information about one of these two factors then information about the other two may lead to a more accurate prediction.

Frequency of occurrence of high risk injuries. When the epilepsy rates for various combinations of factors are displayed beside the frequency with which these combinations in fact occur it becomes clear that highly epileptogenic injuries are relatively rare (Fig. 14). Only about 4% of compound depressed fractures have a late epilepsy risk exceeding 40%. The risk is less than 10% in more than half the patients, and less than 5% in about 40% of fractures. It is therefore possible to reassure many patients with depressed fracture that the risk of late epilepsy is quite small.

Chapter 17

EPILEPSY AFTER INTRACRANIAL
HAEMATOMA

A distinction is drawn between acute and chronic haematomas, although this is seldom done in the few references in the literature to epilepsy after haematoma. Chronic haematomas, evacuated more than 2 weeks after injury, are almost all subdural in site and present such an entirely different problem that it seems proper to deal with them separately. It was noted previously that birth injuries were excluded and very few infantile haematomas appeared in this series (only 5% were under 2 years of age). Acute subdural or intracerebral haematoma almost always implies cortical laceration and contusion whilst extradural haematoma often occurs after mild injury. This is reflected in the different clinical presentation of the latter, which frequently occurs after a lucid interval, the patient having recovered consciousness after injury (or never was unconscious) before signs of cerebral compression developed. Successful surgical treatment depends on rapid evacuation of the clot, and it is therefore of interest to consider the value of epilepsy in the diagnosis of this condition. By contrast patients with acute subdural and intracerebral haematoma are commonly injured more seriously at the outset, and are often already in coma with neurological signs; epilepsy in such a context is neither unexpected nor diagnostically of particular significance. This distinction between intradural and extradural haematomas is less clear than is commonly believed, however. Jamieson and Yelland (1968) drew attention to evidence of intradural pathology in 47% of a series of 167 extradural haematomas. The present series indicates that a number of patients have both extradural and intradural haematomas whilst amongst intradural haematomas there is often a combination of subdural and intracerebral clot, comprising what is sometimes termed "a burst temporal lobe". The difference between extradural and intradural haematomas also makes the significance of late epilepsy different in the two instances; patients surviving after extradural haematoma have commonly made a complete recovery which epilepsy may mar, while survivors from intradural haematomas frequently have fixed neurological deficit and, as in the acute stage, epilepsy is incidental to this problem.

Few reports about acute haematoma even refer to epilepsy and none has analysed its occurrence in detail. When epilepsy is mentioned the time of occurrence is seldom recorded, but as almost all reports are about the acute stage of the condition it is probable that they refer to early epilepsy. For extradural haematoma the incidence would appear to be less than 10%, taking the average for a number of rather small series (17/1). That epilepsy is uncommon is presumably the reason why neither of two recent large series, each of 167 cases, even mentions epilepsy in the course of a very detailed discussion about the symptomatology of this condition (Jamieson and Yelland, 1968; Gallacher and Browder, 1968). In published series of intradural haematomas the rate is somewhat higher (17/16).

17/1a   *Epilepsy associated with extradural haematoma*

Kennedy & Wortis (1936)	$5/17$	29%
McKenzie (1938)	$2/20$	10%
White *et al.* (1948)	$1/9$	11%
Lewin (1949)	$6/26$	23%
Makela (1950)	$0/12$	0%
James & Turner (1951)	$0/36$	0%
McKissock *et al.* (1960b)	$5/125$	4%
Total	$19/245$	8%

17/1b   *Epilepsy associated with acute intradural haematoma*

Subdural		
Kennedy & Wortis (1936)	$10/72$	14%
Gurdjian & Webster (1958)	$29/109$	27%
McKissock *et al.* (1960a)	$10/173$	6%
Jamieson & Yelland (1972)	$62/553$	11%
Intracerebral		
Jamieson & Yelland (1972)	$10/63$	16%
Total	$124/982$	13%

Present Series

In the original Oxford 1,000 there were 58 haematomas, 40% of which were extradural; 362 have been added of which 34% were extradural.

Early epilepsy was significantly more common in those with acute haematoma (17/2), both in adults and children (17/3) and whether or not PTA was prolonged (17/4). The incidence was similar after haematoma in adults and children, including those under 5, and it was not significantly increased by prolonged PTA or when there were focal signs (17/5). Multiple haematomas had only a slightly higher incidence (17/6), but

17/2 *Effect of haematoma on incidence of early epilepsy*

No haematoma	$33/928$	4%
Intracranial haematoma	$112/420$	27%
P	< 0.001	

17/3 *Effect of age and haematoma on incidence of early epilepsy*

	< 16 years		> 16 years	
No haematoma	$8/193$	4%	$25/735$	3%
Intracranial haematoma	$17/68$	25%	$95/352$	27%
P	< 0.001		< 0.001	

17/4 *Effect of PTA and acute haematoma on incidence of early epilepsy*

PTA	< 24 hours		> 24 hours	
No haematoma	$17/711$	2%	$14/130$	11%
Intracranial haematoma	$36/136$	26%	$62/210$	30%
P	< 0.001		< 0.001	

extradural haematoma had a significantly lower epilepsy rate than either solitary subdural or intracerebral haematoma (17/7), or intradural haematomas as a group (including multiple clots) (17/8). In two thirds of cases epilepsy began before evacuation of the haematoma (17/9).

Epilepsy after haematoma was significantly more often delayed beyond 24 hours and only 10% in the first hour after injury (17/10). Both focal and focal motor epilepsy were somewhat more common than after other types of injury (17/11). Early fits were more often repeated after haematoma but status was no more common (17/12).

17/5 *Incidence of early epilepsy after acute intracranial haematoma with various features*

	Feature present		Feature absent		P
< 5 years	$9/28$	32%	$103/392$	26%	NS
> 16 years	$95/352$	27%	$17/68$	25%	NS
PTA > 24 hours	$62/210$	30%	$36/136$	26%	NS
Focal signs	$50/175$	29%	$62/245$	25%	NS

17/6 *Incidence of early epilepsy after single and multiple acute haematomas*

Single	$91/357$	25%
Multiple	$21/63$	33%
P		NS

17/7 *Incidence of early epilepsy with different haematoma site*

Extradural	$15/146$	10%
Subdural	$58/159$	36%
Intracerebral	$18/60$	30%

17/8   *Effect of site of haematoma on incidence of early epilepsy*

Extradural only	$^{15}/_{146}$	10%
Intradural haematoma	$^{97}/_{274}$	35%
P	< 0.001	

17/9   *Early epilepsy and surgery for acute haematoma*

Only before operation	50	56%
Only after	30	34%
Both	9	10%
All before	59	66%
All after	39	44%

17/10   *Time of onset of early epilepsy with acute haematoma*

	First hour		1–24 hours		> 24 hours	
Haematoma 108	11	10%	23	21%	74	69%
No haematoma 107	107	35%	119	37%	95	30%
P	< 0.001		< 0.01		< 0.001	

17/11   *Type of early fit with acute haematoma*

	Focal		Focal motor	
Haematoma 112	70	63%	58	52%
No haematoma 322	173	55%	127	39%
P	NS		NS	

17/12   *Number of fits with acute haematoma*

	% single		% status	
Haematoma	$^{24}/_{110}$	22%	$^{14}/_{110}$	13%
No haematoma	$^{124}/_{320}$	39%	$^{35}/_{320}$	11%
P	< 0.01		NS	

Late Epilepsy

Mortality was high for haematomas, and the number followed for more than a year was only 128. It was shown that these did not differ significantly from the original series (6/7). Late epilepsy was significantly more common after acute intracranial haematoma (17/13), and this was so whether PTA was more or less than 24 hours (17/14). The incidence was significantly higher after intradural haematoma than after extradural (17/15). The epilepsy rate did not differ significantly in patients with various different features (17/16).

17/13   *Effect of acute haematoma on incidence of late epilepsy*

No haematoma	$^{27}/_{854}$	3%
Acute haematoma	$^{45}/_{128}$	35%
P	< 0.001	

17/14   *Effect of acute haematoma and PTA on incidence of late epilepsy*

	< 24 hours PTA		> 24 hours PTA		P
No haematoma	$^{8}/_{146}$	6%	$^{10}/_{94}$	11%	NS
Haematoma	$^{12}/_{47}$	26%	$^{33}/_{79}$	42%	NS
P	< 0.001		< 0.001		

17/15   *Incidence of late epilepsy after single intracranial haematomas in different sites*

Extradural	$^{13}/_{59}$	22%
Intradural	$^{25}/_{56}$	45%
P		< 0.01
Subdural (acute)	$^{14}/_{33}$	42%
Intracerebral	$^{11}/_{23}$	48%
P		NS

(Excluding patients with haematoma in more than one site)

17/16   *Incidence of late epilepsy after haematoma with different features*

Feature	Present		Absent		P
Age < 16 years	$^{7}/_{28}$	25%	$^{38}/_{100}$	38%	NS
PTA > 24 hours	$^{33}/_{79}$	42%	$^{12}/_{47}$	26%	NS
Focal signs	$^{29}/_{73}$	39%	$^{16}/_{55}$	29%	NS
After early epilepsy	$^{9}/_{32}$	28%	$^{36}/_{96}$	38%	NS

There was no difference in the time pattern of onset of late epilepsy after haematoma as compared with other injuries (17/17). The analysis of fits occurring in the first few weeks after injury, at an earlier stage in this study, revealed that subdural haematoma was significantly more common in patients whose first traumatic fit occurred in the second, third and fourth weeks after injury, than when it happened either in the first week or after the end of the first month (17/18). Late epilepsy after haematoma was slightly more often focal but the difference was not significant (17/19); it showed no greater and no lesser tendency to be severe or persistent than epilepsy after other types of injury (17/20).

17/17   *Effect of acute haematoma on onset of late epilepsy*

	<3 months	4–12 months	1–4 years	>4 years
Without haematoma	85	113	105	84
387	22%	29%	27%	22%
With haematoma	12	19	17	6
54	22%	35%	32%	11%
P	NS	NS	NS	NS

17/18   *Frequency of subdural haematoma in patients with epilepsy within 8 weeks of injury*

Time of first fit	% with subdural haematoma	
Week 1	$^{40}/_{273}$ 15%	$\left.\rule{0pt}{2.4em}\right\}$ $P < 0.001$
Weeks 2, 3, 4	$^{13}/_{33}$ 39%	
Weeks 5–8	$^{4}/_{33}$ 12%	$\left.\rule{0pt}{1.4em}\right\}$ $P < 0.02$

17/19   *Frequency of focal late epilepsy after haematoma*

Without haematoma	$^{144}/_{388}$	37%
With acute haematoma	$^{31}/_{67}$	46%
P	NS	

17/20   *Severity of late epilepsy after haematoma*

	% with >1 fit/month		% with remission	
No haematoma	$^{103}/_{275}$	37%	$^{61}/_{175}$	22%
After haematoma	$^{15}/_{52}$	28%	$^{20}/_{52}$	38%
P	NS		< 0.02	

Chapter 18

ELECTROENCEPHALOGRAPHY

The literature on the relationship between EEG abnormalities at various times after head injury, and between EEG and traumatic epilepsy, is now voluminous. Twenty years or so ago there were many claims for the value of EEG as a prognostic guide in traumatic epilepsy but in the last 10 years there has been increasing doubt cast on its usefulness in practice. The first edition of this monograph in 1962 struck one of the early notes of caution. Since then Walton (1963) has concluded that it is wiser to base prognosis solely on clinical grounds and Courjon (1969) formed the opinion that positive evaluation of the risk of late epilepsy could not be based on the EEG. More recently Terespolsky (1972), reviewing the whole field of post-traumatic epilepsy, has supported these views and warned against over-zealous interpretation of results of EEG records. The analysis of the present results adds more weight to this view. In these circumstances a detailed review of the literature seems out of place, and only a few key papers will be mentioned.

One possible reason for the disparity between different reports lies in the widely varying degrees of expertise and styles which exist in recording and interpreting EEG results, together with different indications for the use of this investigation. In the present study of hospital admissions EEGs were not done in the acute stages as a routine, and in many instances it was the suspicion of a complication or failure to recover rapidly which led to records being taken. By contrast one study reported 200 head injuries with EEG records taken in the first aid station of an industrial organisation, half the patients having been so trivially injured that they returned to work next day (Dow *et al.*, 1945).

Head Injury and the EEG

A much quoted study was that of Williams (1941a) who found three main abnormalities in 74 cases of head injury with records during the first 20 days after injury. These were widespread slow waves, suppression of normal frequencies and outbursts of high voltage slow waves. The latter was regarded as epileptic in nature and when persisting for more than 8 days were invariably associated with clinical epilepsy. This time relation is interesting in the light of the frequency of epilepsy within the first week after injury, which the present study has revealed.

Published series of EEG findings at long intervals after injury are usually based on severe injuries still under observation, or on milder cases returning with persisting symptoms. It is not surprising that a high proportion of such records should be abnormal. In following patients until they became symptom-free (Williams, 1941b) found a steady decline in the number of abnormal records between the 4th and 10th week after injury; there was then an increased proportion of abnormal records until the 6th month, which continued after a temporary decline until the 12th month. By this time 55% of records were abnormal and a year later 47% were still abnormal. If PTA had been prolonged the record was more likely to remain abnormal.

In the series of Heppenstall and Hill (1943) EEG abnormalities bore no relation to the time since injury but were commoner if age at injury was less than 20 years. Focal abnormalities were more frequent when there had been prolonged PTA, if there was post-traumatic epilepsy or any other organic post-traumatic syndrome. They were therefore taken as evidence of an acquired cerebral lesion; in contrast diffuse abnormalities, which showed no relation to these factors, were thought to indicate a constitutional disorder. Greenblatt (1943) also found no relationship between either length of PTA or interval since injury and the incidence of diffuse abnormality; he therefore suspected that these abnormalities had little to do with the injury. He found support for this view in a comparison of groups of patients with similar symptomatology with and without a preceding head injury; the number of abnormal records was almost exactly the same in the two series. Courjon (1969) found diffuse abnormalities much commoner in children and adolescents; these usually did not appear in the first few days but in the first few weeks after injury, and commonly disappeared within 6 months.

Traumatic Epilepsy and the EEG

There were abnormal records in 65% of 48 patients with epilepsy reported by Williams (1941b). In 42% the record was a frankly epileptic one resembling that seen in constitutional idiopathic epilepsy. However, records resembling those of constitutional epilepsy were rare in the experience of Jasper and Penfield (1943), only 9 in a series of 86 cases. Local random spikes or sharp waves in a background of delta activity was the usual finding and in 70% a single local unilateral focus was found. In 23%, however, homologous contralateral activity was observed, usually associated with temporal or inferior frontal foci. These are areas commonly damaged bilaterally in closed injuries, and bilateral abnormality may just as well reflect damage on both sides as the activation of normal cortex on one side by injury on the other.

The significance of diffuse and persisting abnormalities of EEG which resemble those of constitutional epilepsy is not clear. They may in fact indicate that the patient had an abnormal record before injury. On the other hand diffuse damage can be caused by acceleration-deceleration injury. Brain stem damage might also be responsible for bilateral changes in the electrical activity of the cortex. Williams (1950) postulated that a focal brain lesion might induce electrical abnormalities which could be delayed for 3-6 months after injury but could then be permanent. He considered that early excision of the damaged area of brain might prevent this development, but that once a diffuse abnormality was established removal of the local lesion would not alter the situation. There may be a parallel with the two quite different kinds of EEG abnormality which have been reported in the recovery period after brain abscess (Northcroft and Wyke, 1957). One consisted of bilateral synchronous paroxysms independent of the site of the abscess, which was regarded as the activation of an inherent convulsive disposition; the record of these patients, who usually had only generalised fits, often reverted to normal over a period of months. The other abnormality was focal paroxysmal activity associated with focal fits, and this usually persisted.

Focal dysrhythmias were excessively rare in Phillips (1954) series of closed injuries; his data was confined to data taken soon after injury in patients with focal signs or depressed fracture, particularly when these had been followed by focal fits. On the other hand Vitale et al. (1953), in patients with traumatic epilepsy, found a temporary focus in a fifth of cases suffering generalised fits and in three quarters of those with temporal lobe epilepsy.

Courjon (1969) followed over 100 patients from the time of injury until late epilepsy appeared. In 40% the EEG record became normal during the incubation period for late epilepsy, whilst abnormalities were often persistent for years in patients who never developed epilepsy. At the time of onset of late epilepsy 25% of patients had normal records. A change from focal slow activity to focal spikes was liable to be associated with the development of late epilepsy.

Present Series

There are obvious limitations when it comes to interpreting EEG records which have accumulated over several years and from several different centres. A simple classification has therefore been adopted which recognises only diffuse or local abnormalities; some patients have both types of abnormality and therefore the totals in tables indicating all patients with diffuse, and all patients with local abnormalities, results in a total larger than the number of the records or of the patients. In the first edition some records were regarded as showing suspected or definite epileptic activity. In discussions since then it has become clear that no consensus exists about what type of abnormality (if any) should be regarded as indicative of epileptic activity and therefore this category of abnormality has not been used.

There is a wide variety in the time after injury when records were taken, because no formal scheme was in operation for undertaking EEGs at regular intervals after injury in the centres from which these cases were collected; about a third of the patients had serial records.

Many previous reports quote the percentage of patients with or without epilepsy who have abnormal records but without having indicated the time after injury when the record was taken. It is clear from the literature, and it has been confirmed by analysis of present data, that abnormalities in the early stages after head injury are very common and that these frequently resolve in the first few weeks. *Per contra* records which are taken only after late epilepsy has been established, a year or two after injury, may show abnormalities in quite a high proportion; but this does not necessarily mean that EEG at an earlier stage would have proved useful in predicting that epilepsy would develop. In the following discussion of data from the present study considerable emphasis is placed on the relationship between EEG abnormalities and the time after injury when the record was taken. The crucial task for the clinician is to recognise which EEG changes after the first three weeks or so may be associated with the subsequent development of epilepsy. In the following tables the group of patients categorised as "with late epilepsy" does not imply that the epilepsy has necessarily already developed at the time when the EEG was recorded.

Over 1,000 records were taken on 722 patients, 204 of whom had more than one record. There were 391 *records* from patients with late, and 303 from those with early, epilepsy; 300 *patients* with late epilepsy, and 180 with early epilepsy had an EEG record at some time after injury. Analysis of records and of patients is undertaken separately, patients with serial records appearing more than once in the records section.

Within the first week after injury over 80% of records showed some abnormality, local changes being almost twice as common as diffuse. The overall abnormality rate declined over the first few months to about 60% and then remained at about that level (18/1). However, the local abnormalities improved much more consistently with time after injury, suggesting that these were related to recent brain damage. Presumably the diffuse abnormalities, which improve less with time, reflect constitutional factors. Records from patients who had *early* epilepsy were significantly more often abnormal in the first week than were those without early

18/1   *Abnormalities in all records at different times after injury*

Time after injury	All abnormalities		Diffuse abnormalities		Local abnormalities	
< 8 days	$146/177$	82%	$51/177$	29%	$123/177$	70%
9 days–3 months	$204/284$	72%	$103/284$	36%	$162/284$	57%
4–12 months	$96/151$	64%	$30/151$	20%	$75/151$	50%
1–2 years	$81/128$	63%	$29/128$	23%	$59/128$	46%
> 2 years	$172/266$	65%	$90/266$	34%	$111/266$	42%
< 4 months	$350/461$	76%	$154/461$	33%	$283/461$	62%
> 4 months	$349/545$	64%	$149/545$	27%	$245/545$	45%
P	< 0.001		NS		< 0.001	
< 4 months	$350/461$	76%	$154/461$	33%	$285/461$	62%
4–12 months	$96/151$	64%	$30/151$	20%	$75/151$	50%
P	< 0.01		< 0.01		< 0.01	
4–12 months	$96/151$	64%	$30/151$	20%	$75/151$	50%
> 1 year	$253/394$	64%	$119/394$	30%	$170/394$	43%
P	NS		< 0.02		NS	
< 1 year	$446/612$	73%	$184/612$	30%	$360/612$	59%
> 1 year	$253/394$	64%	$119/394$	30%	$170/394$	43%
P	< 0.01		NS		< 0.01	

epilepsy; this was due to diffuse rather than local abnormalities (18/2). After that, however, there was no difference between those with and without early epilepsy.

18/2a *Abnormalities in records from patients with and without early epilepsy*

| Time after injury | All abnormalities | | | | P |
	No early		With early		
< 8 days	$^{81}/_{104}$	78%	$^{65}/_{73}$	89%	NS
9 days–3 months	$^{128}/_{190}$	67%	$^{76}/_{94}$	80%	< 0.02
4–12 months	$^{66}/_{97}$	68%	$^{30}/_{54}$	56%	NS
1–2 years	$^{53}/_{88}$	60%	$^{28}/_{40}$	70%	NS
> 2 years	$^{143}/_{224}$	64%	$^{29}/_{42}$	69%	NS
< 4 months	$^{209}/_{294}$	71%	$^{141}/_{167}$	84%	< 0.01
> 4 months	$^{262}/_{409}$	64%	$^{87}/_{136}$	64%	NS
P	NS		< 0.001		
< 4 months	$^{209}/_{294}$	71%	$^{141}/_{167}$	84%	NS
4–12 months	$^{66}/_{97}$	68%	$^{30}/_{54}$	56%	NS
P	NS		< 0.001		
4–12 months	$^{66}/_{97}$	68%	$^{30}/_{54}$	56%	NS
> 1 year	$^{196}/_{312}$	63%	$^{57}/_{82}$	70%	NS
P	NS		NS		
< 1 year	$^{275}/_{391}$	70%	$^{171}/_{221}$	77%	NS
> 1 year	$^{196}/_{312}$	63%	$^{57}/_{82}$	70%	NS
P	NS		NS		

18/2b *Abnormalities in records from patients with and without early epilepsy*

Time after injury	Diffuse abnormalities				P
	No early		With early		
< 8 days	$^{21}/_{104}$	20%	$^{30}/_{73}$	41%	< 0.01
9 days–3 months	$^{67}/_{190}$	35%	$^{36}/_{94}$	38%	NS
4–12 months	$^{19}/_{97}$	20%	$^{11}/_{54}$	20%	NS
1–2 years	$^{21}/_{88}$	24%	$^{8}/_{40}$	20%	NS
> 2 years	$^{74}/_{224}$	33%	$^{16}/_{42}$	20%	NS
< 4 months	$^{88}/_{294}$	30%	$^{66}/_{167}$	40%	NS
> 4 months	$^{114}/_{409}$	28%	$^{35}/_{136}$	26%	NS
P	NS		< 0.02		
< 4 months	$^{88}/_{294}$	35%	$^{66}/_{167}$	40%	NS
4–12 months	$^{19}/_{97}$	20%	$^{11}/_{54}$	20%	NS
P	NS		< 0.02		
4–12 months	$^{19}/_{97}$	20%	$^{11}/_{54}$	20%	NS
> 1 year	$^{95}/_{312}$	30%	$^{24}/_{82}$	29%	NS
P	NS		NS		
< 1 year	$^{107}/_{391}$	27%	$^{77}/_{221}$	35%	NS
> 1 year	$^{95}/_{372}$	30%	$^{24}/_{82}$	29%	NS
P	NS		NS		

18/2c   *Abnormalities in records from patients with and without early epilepsy*

Time after injury	Local abnormalities					P
	No early		With early			
< 8 days	$75/104$	72%	$48/73$	66%		NS
9 days–3 months	$103/190$	54%	$59/94$	63%		NS
4–12 months	$50/97$	52%	$25/54$	46%		NS
1–2 years	$38/88$	43%	$21/40$	52%		NS
> 2 years	$89/224$	40%	$22/42$	52%		NS
< 4 months	$178/294$	61%	$107/167$	64%		NS
> 4 months	$177/409$	43%	$68/136$	50%		NS
P	< 0.001		NS			
< 4 months	$178/294$	61%	$107/167$	64%		NS
4–12 months	$50/97$	52%	$25/54$	46%		NS
P	NS		NS			
4–12 months	$50/97$	52%	$25/54$	46%		NS
> 1 year	$127/312$	41%	$43/82$	52%		NS
P	NS		NS			
< 1 year	$228/391$	58%	$132/221$	60%		NS
> 1 year	$127/312$	41%	$43/82$	52%		NS
P	< 0.001		NS			

18/3 *All injuries, all records, any time*

	No late 510		With late 391		P
All abnormalities	$^{349}/_{510}$	68%	$^{282}/_{391}$	72%	NS
Local	$^{266}/_{510}$	52%	$^{193}/_{391}$	49%	NS
Diffuse	$^{142}/_{510}$	28%	$^{128}/_{391}$	33%	NS

When those who did and those who did not have *late* epilepsy were compared no difference was found for all records regardless of time since injury (18/3). More than 2 years after injury records from those with epilepsy were more often abnormal (18/4). This difference was more marked for local than diffuse abnormalities but it reached significance only when *all* abnormalities were compared in the epilepsy and no epilepsy groups. Although a significant difference between epilepsy and no epilepsy groups is seen in all records taken more than 4 months after injury, and also more than a year after injury, this is chiefly because of the contribution made to these groups by those with abnormal records more than 2 years after injury. Moreover the rise in abnormal records at this late stage is largely accounted for by patients who have already developed late epilepsy, so that it does not indicate a predictive role for the EEG. Epileptic activity has not been analysed on the present expanded series for the reasons given previously, but the findings reported in the first edition indicated that epileptic activity (as then defined) was delayed in appearance, occurring twice as often after three months as before this (18/5).

It might be expected that serial records of individual patients might provide more helpful information, even allowing for the well-known variation in records taken on different occasions in patients with any kind of epilepsy. In fact the majority of such patients showed no change in their records, which were either repeatedly abnormal, or less often, always normal (18/6). There was a sizeable number which became normal when they were repeated, largely accounted for by those who had abnormal records in the first week or month after injury. In only 5% of patients did an abnormality develop after a previously normal record, and in half of these the record had been abnormal before it became normal. In 8 of these 12 patients the record was normal at some time in the first year prior to becoming abnormal later. Only half of this small group of patients with records which became secondarily abnormal developed late

18/4a   *Abnormalities in records from patients who do and do not develop late epilepsy*

| Time after injury | All abnormalities | | | | P |
	No late		With late		
< 8 days	$^{98}/_{121}$	81%	$^{15}/_{17}$	88%	NS
9 days–3 months	$^{138}/_{190}$	73%	$^{48}/_{59}$	81%	NS
4–12 months	$^{51}/_{87}$	59%	$^{38}/_{57}$	67%	NS
1–2 years	$^{37}/_{58}$	64%	$^{35}/_{57}$	61%	NS
> 2 years	$^{25}/_{54}$	46%	$^{146}/_{201}$	73%	< 0.001
< 4 months	$^{236}/_{311}$	76%	$^{63}/_{76}$	83%	NS
> 4 months	$^{113}/_{199}$	57%	$^{219}/_{315}$	70%	< 0.01
P	< 0.001		< 0.02		
< 4 months	$^{236}/_{311}$	76%	$^{63}/_{76}$	83%	NS
4–12 months	$^{51}/_{87}$	59%	$^{38}/_{57}$	67%	NS
P	< 0.01		NS		
4–12 months	$^{51}/_{87}$	59%	$^{38}/_{57}$	67%	
> 1 year	$^{62}/_{112}$	55%	$^{181}/_{258}$	70%	< 0.01
P	NS		NS		
< 1 year	$^{287}/_{398}$	72%	$^{101}/_{133}$	76%	NS
> 1 year	$^{62}/_{112}$	55%	$^{181}/_{258}$	70%	< 0.01
P	< 0.001		NS		

epilepsy. Courjon (1969) has commented on the fact that the disappearance of an early abnormality does not guarantee continued normality of the EEG, nor freedom from epilepsy.

18/4b   *Abnormalities in records from patients who do and do not develop late epilepsy*

Time after injury	Diffuse abnormalities				P
	No late		With late		
< 8 days	$^{29}/_{121}$	24%	$^{4}/_{17}$	24%	NS
9 days–3 months	$^{68}/_{190}$	36%	$^{24}/_{59}$	41%	NS
4–12 months	$^{19}/_{87}$	22%	$^{16}/_{57}$	18%	NS
1–2 years	$^{12}/_{58}$	12%	$^{15}/_{57}$	26%	NS
> 2 years	$^{14}/_{54}$	26%	$^{75}/_{201}$	37%	NS
< 4 months	$^{97}/_{311}$	31%	$^{28}/_{76}$	37%	NS
> 4 months	$^{45}/_{199}$	25%	$^{100}/_{315}$	32%	NS
P	NS		NS		
< 4 months	$^{97}/_{311}$	31%	$^{28}/_{76}$	37%	NS
4–12 months	$^{19}/_{87}$	22%	$^{10}/_{57}$	18%	NS
P	NS		< 0.02		
4–12 months	$^{19}/_{87}$	22%	$^{10}/_{57}$	18%	NS
> 1 year	$^{26}/_{112}$	23%	$^{90}/_{258}$	35%	NS
P	NS		< 0.02		
< 1 year	$^{116}/_{398}$	29%	$^{38}/_{133}$	29%	NS
> 1 year	$^{26}/_{112}$	23%	$^{90}/_{258}$	35%	NS
P	NS		NS		

18/4c *Abnormalities in records from patients who do and do not develop late epilepsy*

	Local abnormalities				
Time after injury	No late		With late		P
< 8 days	$78/121$	65%	$13/17$	76%	NS
9 days–3 months	$103/190$	54%	$34/59$	58%	NS
4–12 months	$39/87$	45%	$29/57$	51%	NS
1–2 years	$39/58$	50%	$23/57$	40%	NS
> 2 years	$17/54$	32%	$94/201$	47%	NS
< 4 months	$181/311$	58%	$47/76$	62%	NS
> 4 months	$85/199$	43%	$146/315$	46%	NS
P	< 0.001		< 0.02		
< 4 months	$181/311$	58%	$47/76$	62%	NS
4–12 months	$39/87$	45%	$29/57$	51%	NS
P	NS		NS		
4–12 months	$39/87$	45%	$29/57$	51%	NS
> 1 year	$46/112$	41%	$117/258$	45%	NS
P	NS		NS		
< 1 year	$220/398$	55%	$76/133$	57%	NS
> 1 year	$46/112$	41%	$117/258$	45%	NS
P	< 0.01		NS		

Half of the 184 patients who had at least one record during the first 3 months after injury, and who were followed for more than a year, had at least one normal record during this early period (18/7). Such a normal record was more common in those who did not develop late epilepsy, but for predictive purposes it is important to emphasise that 20% of those who developed late epilepsy had had a normal record within the first 3 months after injury.

In order to discount the probable irrelevance of abnormalities in the very early stages, as a predictive criterion, an analysis was next made of patients who had one or more records taken more than 3 weeks after injury, and taking account only of these later records. In patients who developed late epilepsy this record was more often abnormal, but the difference between the epilepsy and non-epilepsy groups were not striking (18/8). It seemed likely that abnormalities persisting after 3 weeks might show some correlation with those clinical features of injury which are usually taken to reflect a greater degree of brain damage. Indeed abnormal records did prove to be more common in patients with prolonged PTA, with focal signs or with a compound depressed fracture associated with dural tearing (18/9). Now these are all factors which have also been shown to be associated with an increased risk of epilepsy. This suggests that the EEG abnormalities are largely a reflection of increased brain damage, which is already evident from clinical data. To that extent the EEG data may be regarded as largely redundant (see page 160). It is certainly doubtful whether the EEG adds to the discrimination already achieved on the basis of clinical data.

It must be concluded that the EEG does not contribute materially to the problem of predicting late epilepsy in individual patients, even although some trends towards a greater degree of abnormality in the epilepsy group can be detected in large groups of patients. Many patients with persisting EEG abnormalities do not develop epilepsy and even those who develop delayed local spike activity do not necessarily go on to have fits. Of those who do develop epilepsy a quarter never have an abnormal record, a fifth have a normal record within 3 weeks of injury and a third have a normal record at some time or other after the first three weeks. Moreover a number of patients have a normal record at the time when the late epilepsy begins and only develop abnormalities at a later stage, once the traumatic epilepsy is established.

It seems likely that the increased incidence of EEG abnormalities in patients with traumatic epilepsy, as compared with other patients, is largely accounted for by their having more brain damage rather than by the late development of abnormalities. Those concerned with electro-encephalography may protest that what is required is more careful or more

18/5 *Epileptic activity in records after injury*
(first edition data)

< 3 months	$^8/_{41}$	20%
> 3 months	$^{148}/_{342}$	43%
P	< 0.01	

18/6 *Serial records in 204 patients*

Always abnormal	116
Always normal	21
Abnormal becoming normal	63
Normal becoming abnormal	12

(8 patients changed twice)

18/7 *Of patients with at least one EEG in the first 3 months after injury*

$^{79}/_{128}$ (62%) with no late epilepsy

were normal

$^{11}/_{56}$ (20%) with late epilepsy

P < 0.001

18/8a *EEG abnormalities more than 3 weeks after injury*
(patients)

	No early 415		After early 131		P
Only abnormal	244	59%	76	58%	NS
Ever abnormal	260	63%	86	66%	NS
Only abnormal	134	32%	51	39%	NS
Ever normal	171	41%	69	53%	NS

18/8b *EEG abnormalities more than 3 weeks after injury and late epilepsy* (patients)

	No late 216		With late 288		P
Only abnormal	103	48%	197	68%	< 0.001
Ever abnormal	117	54%	206	72%	< 0.001
Only normal	74	34%	79	27%	NS
Ever normal	112	52%	91	32%	< 0.001

18/9 *Features associated with EEGs more than 3 weeks after injury* (patients)

	Only abnormal 320		Only normal 164		P
Early epilepsy	76	24%	30	18%	NS
PTA > 24 hours	151	47%	54	33%	< 0.01
Focal signs	98	31%	35	21%	NS
Compound depressed fracture	152	48%	67	41%	NS
Dura torn	98	31%	28	17%	< 0.01

18/9b

	Ever abnormal 349		Ever normal 230		P
Early epilepsy	85	24%	55	24%	NS
PTA > 24 hours	161	46%	72	31%	< 0.01
Focal signs	104	30%	43	19%	< 0.01
Compound depressed fracture	172	49%	109	47%	NS
Dura torn	110	32%	45	19%	< 0.01

elaborate EEG investigations, including sleep records, or activation techniques. It may well be that certain specialised centres might improve the discriminating ability of the EEG, but it has to be remembered that head injury is a very common condition, occurring in thousands of patients every year, and the majority will not have access to highly specialised centres. What doctors and lawyers have to consider is the practical implications of an EEG done on a random basis in a centre not specially interested or devoted to this topic. The evidence of the present study is that such an EEG adds little if anything to the doctor's ability to predict whether or not epilepsy will develop, a normal record being only marginally reassuring and an abnormal record not necessarily presaging late epilepsy. This accords with the views of Walton (1963), Courjon (1969) and Terespolsky (1972) and can therefore be regarded as a consensus opinion in the present state of knowledge.

Chapter 19

PREDICTION OF LATE EPILEPSY

The results of the present investigation provide a basis for calculating the probability that late epilepsy will develop in individual head injured patients. It has enabled those few factors which are powerful predictors to be identified, whilst at the same time demonstrating that many other features, which might intuitively have been expected to be important, have little connection with the subsequent development of epilepsy. In common with other recent studies involving computer-aided diagnosis this investigation resulted in a reduction in the amount of information required to reach a decision. The statistical basis for this simplification lies in the fact that some of the factors concerned are not independent, so that when all possible variables are taken account of there is a high degree of redundancy; these theoretical considerations have been discussed by Teather (1974) and by Card and Good (1973). Elsewhere Card (1973) has observed that clinicians habitually undervalue the power of the data which is readily available to them, and this has clearly been so in the field of traumatic epilepsy.

This is chiefly because doctors cannot adequately manipulate the data they have, nor do they know the relative value of different items of data (i.e. the weight of evidence). The clinicians' response to his inability to reach a clear decision is usually to acquire more information, although there is evidence that this frequently compounds his confusion. What is required is not more but less data, with the proviso that this data is rationally selected and is efficiently manipulated. Using the computer as a tool, and mathematics as a method, it is now possible to determine the weight of the evidence, and so to choose to collect the data which will be most useful. The paradox is that this use of the complexities of probability statistics and of computerisation ultimately simplifies the process of decision-making at the clinical level.

This is nowhere more evident than in the prediction of late epilepsy, which has now been shown to depend on very few items of information — indeed only three factors significantly increase the incidence of late epilepsy (15/4). These are acute haematoma (31% develop late epilepsy), early epilepsy (25% develop late epilepsy) and depressed fracture (15% develop late epilepsy). When an injury is *not* associated with any of these factors the risk of late epilepsy is only about 1%. Moreover, when there has been either an acute haematoma or early epilepsy then no other feature of the injury makes any significant difference to the risk of late epilepsy; features such as age, focal signs, duration of PTA prove all to be redundant. Not so after depressed fracture, when the incidence of epilepsy may vary from over 60% to less than 4%, according to different combinations of four variables, namely duration of PTA, state of the dura, the occurrence of focal signs and whether there has been early epilepsy. But again there are other features, such as site of fracture and methods of treatment, which have been shown not to influence the incidence of late epilepsy.

Predictions must often be made by doctors who were not associated with the management of the patient immediately after injury. It is of practical interest that the degree of availability of the significant items of information after depressed fracture to such a doctor corresponds with the rank order of the predictive powers of these features. Such a doctor can almost always assess the most valuable predictive datum, which is whether PTA was greater or less than 24 hours, by talking to the patient and the family, without reference to the original notes. Whether or not the dura was torn depends on the information from the surgeon, but this can usually be discovered, especially if enquiries are made soon after injury. Focal neurological signs, the next most useful guide, may not always be recorded or remembered if they were mild and temporary whilst early epilepsy, which is the least important factor after depressed fracture, may well be quite unknown to the patient.

Residual Risk After Fit-free Intervals

When calculations soon after injury indicate a high risk of epilepsy there is a natural concern to know by how much this has been reduced when a certain period has elapsed after injury without a fit having occurred. This can be calculated on the basis of actuarial statistics, as used in the analysis of life tables; this has been described in more detail elsewhere (Jennett, Teather and Bennie, 1973).

The basic formula is $F_0 = S_1 \times F_1$ where

F_0 = probability (p) that patient will remain free of epilepsy
S_1 = probability that he will have no fits in the first year
F_0 = probability that he will remain free after one year.

It is possible to substitute appropriately from the data available in the present study.

$F_0 = 1 - R_0$, where R_0 is the original risk — the predicted probability of epilepsy as calculated one week after injury.

$S_1 = 1 - L_1$, where L_1 is the probability that a patient with that type of injury will develop epilepsy during the first year.

This in turn is derived from O_1, the proportion of patients with late epilepsy after that type of injury whose fits begin in the first year (see Chapter 12). The formula is $L_1 = R_0 \times O_1$.

$F_0 = 1 - R_1$, where R_1 is the residual risk one year after injury, no late fits having so far developed.

The original formula $F_0 = S_1 \times F_1$ becomes $(I - R_0) = (I - L_1) \times (I - R_1)$

$$\text{therefore} \quad R_1 = I - \frac{(I - R_0)}{(I - L_1)}$$

The amount by which the original risk is reduced depends on the proportion of late epilepsy patients with that particular injury whose epilepsy begins in the first year (O_1). Because this varies with the type of injury no constant can be given by which to calculate R_1 from R_0 for all injuries. Consider two types of injury A and B with a similar original risk of 40% late epilepsy ($R_0 = 0.4$). Let O_{IA} be 0.25 (25% of late epilepsy begins within a year), and O_{IB} be 0.75. Then L_{IA} will be $0.4 \times 0.25 = 0.1$ whilst $L_{IB} = 0.4 \times 0.75 = 0.3$.

For injury A:

$$R_1 = I - \frac{I - 0.4}{I - 0.1} = I - 0.66 = 0.34$$

For injury B:

$$R_1 = I - \frac{I - 0.4}{I - 0.3} = I - 0.86 = 0.24$$

The original risk of 40% late epilepsy has fallen at one year to 34% for injury A, and to 24% for injury B. Examples for actual risks in this study are set out in 19/1.

Notice that the fit-free interval referred to here is an interval beginning one week after injury, no late fits having developed at all — it does not apply to a fit-free interval once late epilepsy has occurred. As explained in Chapter 10 there is no way of calculating the likelihood of recurrence once late epilepsy has developed even when there has been a remission of a year or more.

Prophylactic Anticonvulsant Medication

An important reason for wishing to calculate the original and residual risk of late epilepsy in individual patients is in order to reach a decision about

19/1   *Reduction of risk if no late epilepsy in first year, for various initial risks*

Type of injury	Initial risk	Residual risk (at one year)
Early epilepsy	28%	10%
Haematoma	35%	19%
Depressed fracture*	15%	9%
	20%	12%
	25%	15%
	30%	19%
	35%	22%
	40%	26%
	45%	30%
	50%	34%
	55%	39%
	60%	45%
	65%	50%
	70%	55%

* After various levels of initial risk, assuming that proportion beginning in first year (O_1) is the same; if early epilepsy has occurred then O_1 is higher, so that the residual risk (if no late epilepsy in first year after injury) is *lower* than shown here.

recommending anticonvulsant drugs. A recent review of the literature has adduced a considerable amount of experimental and clinical evidence which indicates that anticonvulsant medication can be effective in reducing the incidence of post-traumatic epilepsy (Rapport and Penry, 1972). These same authors subsequently investigated the practice of over 1,000 American neurosurgeons in regard to prescribing anticonvulsants after head injury (Rapport and Penry, 1973). Some 40% of the neurosurgeons questioned did not use prophylactic anticonvulsants routinely, a third of them because they were uncertain of the indications and 14% because they considered the incidence of epilepsy to be too low after non-missile injuries to justify routine drug prophylaxis. Rapport and Penry expressed concern that, in spite of the evidence that anticonvulsants were effective, 40% of surgeons were failing to protect their head injured patients with drugs; they estimated that some 100,000 Americans each year might suffer epilepsy because they had been denied this therapy. The prevailing reason for the reluctance to prescribe prophylactic drugs appears to have been uncertainty about the actual risk of epilepsy in individual patients — in their own words "even the criteria for identifying which head injured patients are most likely to develop post-traumatic seizures are unclear".

This excuse is no longer valid, because the present investigation has indicated what risk of epilepsy applies after various types of injury. What clinicians must now decide is the level of risk which they consider high enough to justify the prescription of anticonvulsant drugs. It would then be rational to treat all patients whose calculated original risk is above that level; and to continue treatment until the residual risk falls below that level. What level of risk justifies prophylactic anticonvulsant drugs depends on many factors, the circumstances of the individual patient being the most important. The majority of head injured patients are young and their whole future may depend on decisions made following their injury. The possibility of epilepsy may affect career choice, or even their continuation in a job for which they are already trained. In this regard doctors should not underestimate the serious consequences of even a single fit, under certain circumstances. Although the social stigma of epilepsy is much less than it used to be there are still considerable restrictions of choice on the individual who is known to have had a fit and who is therefore judged likely to have another. Car driving is perhaps the activity most often affected by the risk of epilepsy; but it is fortunate that the law in many countries no longer regards the fact that a driver is taking anticonvulsants as *ipso facto* evidence that he is (in the present tense) suffering from epilepsy, and is therefore ineligible to drive. This should remove one of the reasons for the reluctance to prescribe drugs for patients who have never had a fit (and may never have one), namely the fear that the discovery that he is taking anticonvulsants might be disadvantageous to him.

In only a limited sample of the patient population in the present study was information available about anticonvulsant prescribing soon after injury. As there was no formal code of practice in force in any of the centres involved at the time of data collection this gives some indication of the practice of a considerable number of neurosurgeons over a period of some years. This seems to have been very similar to the current practice in the U.S.A., as reported by Rapport and Penry. Although cases available for study of anticonvulsant prescribing were all in relatively high risk categories (having had either early epilepsy, depressed fracture or acute intracranial haematoma), only 16% had ever had anticonvulsants prescribed. This figure corresponds to the 14% of American neurosurgeons whose practice it was to give anticonvulsants routinely to all head injured patients. However, in the present series, prophylactic anticonvulsants were more often prescribed for those patients who did eventually develop late epilepsy (19/2) and for those who suffered different types of injury which this study has shown to be associated with a high risk (19/3). Only 6% of the patients in the present study had medication for more than 12 months which represents 36% of those who were given anticonvulsants (19/4). In the American study only 176 surgeons declared how long they usually continued drug treatment; 40% did so for one year which again suggests a similar practice to that revealed by the present study.

19/2 *Frequency of initial prescription of anticonvulsants*

All cases	$235/1484$	35%
No late epilepsy	$171/1272$	13%
Late epilepsy (eventually)	$64/212$	30%

19/3 *Anticonvulsants after depressed fracture*

	Closed (45)		Compound dura intact (205)		Compound dura torn (218)	
Any at all	6	13%	44	21%	84	39%
For > 12 months	1	2%	14	7%	43	20%

19/4 *Frequency and duration of anticonvulsant treatment*

Duration of treatment	Of all cases		Of cases given drugs
< 3 months	95	6%	41%
4–12 months	55	4%	23%
> 12 months	85	6%	36%

No attempt was made to determine the efficacy of anticonvulsant therapy, whether given prophylactically or after epilepsy itself. To do so requires a rigorously planned study with frequent checks that the drugs being prescribed are in fact taken regularly (Penry, 1973). Formal trials of prophylactic anticonvulsant medication after head injury are currently in progress (Penry, 1974) and it is to be hoped that when these are published it may be possible to formulate recommendations for the future. It is the view of Rapport and Penry (1973) that to be maximally effective prophylaxis should be initiated immediately after injury because by this means it may be possible to prevent the development of an epileptiform focus.

If controlled trials do support this view then it will be more important than ever to have soundly based criteria for predicting which patients are at risk from late epilepsy. Whilst most analyses presented in this book will be useful for this purpose the predictive value of early epilepsy may be affected to some extent, if it becomes normal practice to administer effective doses of anticonvulsants soon after injury to a substantial proportion of head injuries. Almost a third of early fits begin within an hour of injury, almost two thirds within 24 hours. In many instances, moreover, the injury has been relatively mild and in some the first fit has already occurred before hospitalisation. When it is remembered that high doses of anticonvulsants would have to be administered parentally before effective blood levels are reached, it seems unlikely that a substantial number of first day fits after milder injuries would in practice be suppressed. Moreover, it is patients who are otherwise not predisposed to late epilepsy by reason of intracranial haematoma or certain types of depressed fracture that the occurrence of a fit in the first week is of such importance in indicating the likelihood of late epilepsy — and these are the patients least likely to be given early prophylactic anticonvulsants, if such should become common practice. Whatever conclusions result from the current investigations into the prophylaxis of traumatic epilepsy, it seems likely that there will be a group of patients in whom the risk of late epilepsy, as judged immediately after injury, is not high enough to warrant anticonvulsants until or unless they develop a fit during the first week. In such instances the situation should be revised at the end of the first week; if such patients were to be given drugs immediately after injury then the absence of fits in the first week would not be of prognostic value — at least the data presented from the present study would not apply.

Chapter 20

CONCLUSIONS

Early Epilepsy

Identity of Early Epilepsy

1. Epilepsy occurs much more often in the first week after injury than in any of the next 7 weeks (8/2, p. 29).

2. Focal motor fits are more common in the first week, when temporal lobe attacks never occur (8/4, p. 30).

3. First week epilepsy recurs in the future significantly less often than epilepsy beginning in the next few weeks (8/5, p. 31).

4. Factors affecting the incidence of early and of late epilepsy are different (8/7, 8/8, p. 32, 3)

Incidence of Early Epilepsy

1. At least one fit occurred during the first week after injury in 5% of an unselected group of head injuries.

2. Epilepsy occurred as frequently in adults as in the whole group of children under 16; it was more common under the age of 5 (9/2, p. 36).

3. After injuries with less than 24 hours PTA, or without fracture, epilepsy was more common in children than in adults (9/4, p. 38).

4. Epilepsy rarely followed a trivial injury except in children under 5 (9/7, p. 39).

5. Injuries associated with more than 24 hours PTA were more often followed by epilepsy (9/8, p. 40).

6. This effect of prolonged PTA was significant only in adults, and in patients (regardless of age) with no depressed fracture or haematoma (9/15, p. 43).

7. A linear fracture, regardless of site, increased the incidence of early epilepsy (9/16, p. 44).

8. Depressed fracture was more often followed by epilepsy; this association was less marked in children than in adults, and was not seen at all after prolonged PTA nor when there were focal signs (9/19, p. 45).

9. When there was a depressed fracture the incidence of epilepsy was unaffected by any other features of injury (16/6, p. 103).

10. Acute intracranial haematoma carried a high risk of early epilepsy (9/20, p. 45).

11. Epilepsy was more common after intradural than extradural haematoma (17/8, p. 140).

12. When there was a haematoma the incidence of epilepsy was not affected by any other features of injury (17/5, p. 139).

13. Neurological signs increased the incidence of early epilepsy, regardless of age and the duration of PTA (9/24, p. 47).

14. If the signs were focal the incidence of early epilepsy was still further increased (9/22, p. 46); after depressed fracture or intracranial haematoma, however, focal signs did not add to the already increased incidence of early epilepsy (9/23, p. 46).

15. Early epilepsy was more frequent in patients with subarachnoid haemorrhage, except when there was already a high rate due to prolonged PTA or fracture (9/25, p. 48).

Character of Early Epilepsy

1. More than half the patients had some fits which were recognisably focal in onset, three-quarters of these being focal motor attacks (10/1, p. 50).

2. Focal attacks were somewhat more common with haematoma but not after depressed fracture (10/4, p. 52).

3. Focal attacks were somewhat more common when PTA exceeded 24 hours (10/3, p. 52).

4. The first early fit occurred within 24 hours of injury in half the cases, and in half of these it was within an hour of injury (10/5, p. 53).

5. Fits were more common in the first hour if aged < 16 years (10/5, p. 53); if PTA < 24 hours (10/6, p. 54); if there is depressed fracture or there is not a haematoma (10/9, p. 55).

6. Epilepsy was more often delayed beyond the first day in adults (10/5, p. 53; if PTA < 24 hours (10/6, 7, 8, p. 54); if there is a haematoma or is not a depressed fracture (10/9, p. 55).

7. Two thirds of patients had more than one early seizure (10/10, p. 56).

8. Repeated fits were more commonly focal and more often began more than 24 hours after injury (10/14, p. 58).

9. Status epilepticus developed in 10% of cases, but was more common under the age of 5 (10/10, p. 56).

10. Fits after depressed fracture more often began in the first hour and less often after 24 hours; attacks were more often single (10/9, 10/12, pp. 55, 9).

11. Fits after intracranial haematoma seldom occurred in the first hour and were more often delayed after 24 hours; repeated attacks were more common (10/9, 10/12, pp. 55, 7).

Significance of Early Epilepsy

Indication of Acute Intracranial Haematoma (p. 60)

1. Less than 2% of patients proved to be developing an extradural haematoma at the time of their first fit.

2. Even early epilepsy after injury with no amnesia was only occasionally associated with acute haematoma.

3. A fit was never the only or the first sign of a developing intracranial haematoma.

4. The occurrence of an early fit is therefore insufficient evidence for suspecting an intracranial haematoma, unless there are other signs of this complication.

Mortality (p. 61)

1. The increased mortality rate associated with early epilepsy is almost wholly due to patients with acute intracranial haematoma.

2. Status epilepticus carries the risk of death or permanent brain damage, especially in young children.

Pre-disposition to Late Traumatic Epilepsy (pp. 62-6)

1. Late epilepsy occurred significantly more often when there had been early epilepsy (11/1, 2, pp. 62, 3).

2. This increased risk of late epilepsy was similar at all ages, and whatever the features of injury; it was somewhat less when PTA was less than 24 hours and more marked with prolonged PTA (11/4, p. 64).

3. Late epilepsy after early was just as frequent in the absence of depressed fracture or intracranial haematoma, and was equally common after trivial injuries (11/5, 11/6, p. 65).

4. The incidence of late epilepsy was unaffected by the type, time or number of the early fits (11/7, 11/8, 11/9, pp. 65, 6)

5. Focal early epilepsy in children was the only kind of early epilepsy which did not significantly increase the risk of late epilepsy (11/6, p. 66).

Late Epilepsy

Incidence of Late Epilepsy

1. The overall risk of late epilepsy for an unselected series of head injuries admitted to hospital has been calculated as being 5%.

2. This risk was significantly increased by each of three factors — acute haematoma (31% late epilepsy), early epilepsy (25% late epilepsy) and depressed fracture (15% late epilepsy) (15/4, p. 92).

3. For injuries with none of these features the risk of epilepsy is about 1% (15/10, p. 95).

4. When there had been an acute haematoma or early epilepsy, the incidence of late epilepsy was not further influenced by other features of the injury (17/16, 11/4, pp. 142, 64).

5. After depressed fracture the risk of epilepsy varied from over 50% to less than 4%, according to various other features (Fig. 12, p. 135).

6. No consistent correlation was found between EEG abnormalities in the first year after injury and the development of late epilepsy (18/4, pp. 153-5).

Varying Risk of Late Epilepsy After Depressed Fracture

1. *Children* under 16 years were less liable to develop late epilepsy after depressed fracture than were adults (16/4, p. 000).

2. With *PTA over 24 hours* late epilepsy occurred in a third of depressed fractures (16/19, p. 109); this rate was doubled when there had been early epilepsy (16/42, p. 124), but was not significantly increased by dural tearing or by focal signs (16/44, 5, p. 125).

3. When there had been *early epilepsy,* late epilepsy developed in a quarter of depressed fractures (16/21, p. 110); this rate was increased when PTA > 24 hours (16/42, p. 123) or dura was torn (16/46, p. 125) but not by focal signs (16/47, p. 126).

4. *Focal neurological signs* were associated with a late epilepsy in more than a quarter of depressed fractures (16/27, p. 117); this rate was increased by dural tearing (16/43, p. 124) and by PTA > 24 hours (16/44, p. 125), but not by early epilepsy (16/47, p. 126).

5. Compound depressed fractures with *dural tearing* were followed by late epilepsy in a quarter of cases (16/34, p. 119); the rate was doubled when there were focal signs (16/43, p. 124) or PTA > 24 hours (16/45, p. 125), but not significantly increased by early epilepsy (16/46, p. 125).

6. Factors which did *not* affect the incidence of late epilepsy after depressed fracture, were site of fracture, whether or not the fracture was elevated, and whether, after elevation, bone fragments were removed or replaced.

Character of Late Epilepsy

1. Rather more than half the cases have their fits within a year of injury (excluding cases in the first week) (12/1, p. 69).

2. Late epilepsy in adults more often began in the first year (12/9, p. 73).

3. One patient in 5 with traumatic epilepsy had the first fit more than 4 years after injury (12/4, p. 71).

4. When there had been early epilepsy then late epilepsy more often began in the first year and was less often delayed for more than 4 years (12/12, p. 74).

5. After depressed fracture epilepsy more often began after the first year (12/13, p. 74); haematoma did not influence the time of onset of late epilepsy.

6. Some focal features were found in 40% of patients; temporal lobe seizures occurred in a fifth of cases (13/2, p. 77).

7. The type of complications did not affect the type of fit, except that focal late epilepsy was more common when there had been early epilepsy (13/3, p. 77).

8. More than a third of patients continued to have frequent fits, whilst a quarter had a remission of 2 years or more without fits (14/4, p. 84).

9. When epilepsy began after 4 years fits were more likely to be frequent and remission was less likely (14/5, p. 85).

10. Focal and non-focal epilepsy were equally likely to persist but temporal lobe seizures had a higher persistence rate (14/7, p. 86).

REFERENCES

Ascroft, P. B. (1941). Traumatic epilepsy after gunshot wounds of the head. *Brit. Med. J.* i, 739.

Birkmayer, W. (1949). Zur Frage der traumatischen epilepsie. *Schweiz, Arch. f. Neurol. u. Psychiat.* **63**, 98.

Braakman, R. (1972). Depressed skull fracture; data, treatment and follow-up in 225 consecutive cases. *J. Neurol. Neurosurg. Psychiat.*, **35**, 395.

Brock, S. (1950). "Injuries of Skull, Brain and Spinal Cord". Williams, Wilkins, Baltimore.

Card, W. I. (1973). The computing approach to clinical diagnosis. *Proc. Roy. Soc. Lond. B* **184**, 421.

Card, W. I. and Good, I. J. (1973). "The Mathematical Structure of Clinical Medicine". Edinburgh: University Press.

Caveness, W. F. (1963). Onset and cessation of fits following cranicerebral trauma. *J. Neurosurg.* **20**, 570.

Caveness, W. F. (1962). Incidence of post-traumatic epilepsy in Korean veterans as compared with those from World War I and World War II. *J. Neurosurg.* **19**, 122.

Caveness, W. F. (1964). "Neurological Surgery of Trauma". A. N. Meirowsky, Surgeon General's Dept., Washington. Chapter 21. Clinical manifestations.

Caveness, W. F. and Liss, H. R. (1961). Incidence of post-traumatic epilepsy. *Epilepsia,* **2**, 123.

Cawthorne, T. (1952). Vertigo. *Brit. Med. J.* ii, 931.

Courjon, J. A. (1969). "Post-traumatic Epilepsy in Electroclinical Practice". In: Walker, A. E., Caveness, W. F., Critchley, M. (eds.). The late effects of head injury. Thomas, Springfield.

Credner, L. (1930). Klinische und soziale Auswirkungen von Hirn-schadigungen. *Z. ges. Neurol. Psychiat.* **126**, 721.

Denny-Brown, D. (1943). Clinical aspects of traumatic epilepsy. *Amer. J. Psychiat.* **100**, 585.

Denny-Brown, D. (1941). Delayed collapse after head injury. *Lancet* i, 371.

Dow, R. S., Ulett, G. and Roof, J. (1945). Electroencephalographic studies in head injuries. *J. Neurosurg.* **2**, 154.

Elvidge, A. P. (1950). In "Injuries of Brain and Spinal Cord", Brock B. (q.v.)

English, T. C. (1904). The after effects of head injury. *Lancet* i, 632.

Erculei, F. and Walker, A. E. (1963). Post-traumatic epilepsy and early cranioplasty, *J. Neurosurg.* **20**, 1085.

Evans, J. H. (1962). Post-traumatic epilepsy. *Neurol.* **12**, 662.

Evans, J. H. (1963). The significance of early post-traumatic epilepsy. *Neurol.* **13**, 207.

Feinberg, P. "Epilepsie u. Trauma". Oberholzer, Zurich.

Freeman, W. (1953). Hazards of lobotomy; a study of 2000 operations. *J. Amer. Med. Ass.* **152**, 487.

Garland, H. G. (1942). Discussion on traumatic epilepsy. *Proc. Roy. Soc. Med.* **35**, 773.

Gallacher, J. P. and Browder, E. J. (1968). Extradural haematoma. Experience with 167 patients. *J. Neurosurg.* **29**, 1.

Garland, H. G. and Phillips, W. (1953). Medicine, Macmillan, London.

Glaser, M. A. and Schafer, F. P. (1945). Depressed fractures of the skull, their surgery, sequelae and disability. *J. Neurosurg.* **2**, 140.

Gowers, W. R. (1903). "Borderlands of Epilepsy". Churchill, London.

Grand, W. (1974). The significance of post-traumatic status epilepticus in childhood. *J. Neurol. Neurosurg. Psychiat.* **37**, 178.

Greenblatt, M. (1943). The EEG in late post-traumatic cases. *Amer. J. Psychiat.* **100**, 378.

Groat, R. A., Windle, W. F. and Magoun, H. W. (1945). Functional and structural changes in the monkey's brain during and after concussion. *J. Neurosurg.* **2**, 26.

Gurdjian, E. S. and Webster, J. E. (1958). Head injuries. Little, Brown and Co. Boston, U.S.A.

Hendrick, E. B. and Harris, L. (1968). Post-traumatic epilepsy in children. *Journal of Trauma.* **8**, 547.

Heppenstall, M. E. and Hill, D. (1943). EEG in chronic post-traumatic syndromes. *Lancet,* i, 261.

Hyslop, G. H. (1950). Seizures, head injuries and litigants. *Arch. Neurol. Psychiat. (Chicago)* **64**, 736.

James, T. G. I. and Turner, E. A. (1951). Traumatic intracranial haematoma. *Lancet* ii, 45.

Jamieson, K. G. and Yelland, J. D. N. (1968). Extradural haematoma. Report of 167 cases. *J. Neurosurg.* **29**, 1.

Jamieson, K. G. and Yelland, J. D. N. (1972). Traumatic intracerebral haematoma. Report of 63 surgically treated cases. *J. Neurosurg.* **37** 528.

Jamieson, K. G. and Yelland, J. D. N. (1972). Depressed skull fractures in Australia. *J. Neurosurg.* **37**, 150.

Jamieson, K. G. and Yelland, J. D. N. (1972). Surgically treated traumatic subdural haematoma. *J. Neurosurg.* **37**, 137.

Jasper, H. (1954). See Penfield and Jasper.

Jasper, H. and Penfield, W. (1943). Electroencephalograms in post-traumatic epilepsy: pre-operative and post-operative studies. *Amer. J. Psychiat.* **100**, 365.

Jennett, W. B. (1969). Early traumatic epilepsy. *Lancet* i, 1023.

Jennett, B. (1972). Epilepsy after non-missile head injuries. *Scot. Med. J.* **18**, 18-13.

Jennett, B. (1974). Epilepsy after depressed skull fracture. *J. Neurosurg.* **41**, 208.

Jennett, B. (1974). Early traumatic epilepsy. *Arch. Neurol.* **30**, 394.

Jennett, W. B. and Lewin, W. S. (1960). Traumatic epilepsy after closed head injuries. *J. Neurol. Neurosurg. Psychiat.* **23**, 295.

Jennett, B. and Miller, J. D. (1972). Infection after depressed fracture of the skull. *J. Neurosurg.* **36**, 333.

Jennett, B., Teather, D. and Bennie, S. (1973). Epilepsy after head injury — residual risk after varying fit-free intervals since injury. *Lancet* **2**, 652.

Kennedy, F. and Wortis, H. (1936). "Acute" subdural haematoma and acute epidural haemorrhage; study of 72 cases of haematoma and 17 cases of haemorrhage. *Surg. Gynec. Obstet.* **63**, 732.

Klotz, M. (1955). Incidence of seizures with EEG findings in prefrontal lobotomy. *Arch. Neurol Psychiat. (Chicago)* **74**, 144.

Kriss, F. C., Taren, J. A. and Kahn, E. A. (1969). Primary repair of compound skull fractures by replacement of bone fragments. *J. Neurosurg.* **30**, 698.

Lewin, W. S. (1949). Acute subdural and extradural haematoma in closed head injuries. *Ann. Roy. Coll. Surg. Engl.* **5**, 240.

Lishman, A. (1968). Brain damage in relation to disability after head injury. *Brit. J. Psychiat.* **114**, 373.

McKenzie, K. G. (1938). Extradural haemorrhage. *Brit. J. Surg.* **26**, 346.

McKissock, W., Richardson, A. and Bloom, W. H. (1960a). Subdural haematoma. *Lancet* i, 1365.

McKissock, W., Taylor, J. and Bloom, W. H. (1960b). Extradural haematoma. *Lancet* ii, 167.

Makela, T. (1950). *Ann. Chir. Gyn. Fenn.* **39**, 126.

Malling, K. (1953). *Acta Psychiat.* **8**, 39.

Miller, J. D. and Jennett, W. B. (1968). Complications of depressed skull fracture. *Lancet* **2**, 991.

Mock, H. E. (1950). Skull fractures and brain injuries. Wm. Wilkins, Baltimore, U.S.A.

Muskens, L. J. J. (1928). Epilepsy. Wm. Wood, New York, U.S.A.

Munro, D. (1938). "Craniocerebral Injuries". Oxford Univ. Press. New York, U.S.A.

Northcroft, G. B. and Wyke, B. D. (1957). Seizures following surgical treatment of intracranial abscesses. A clinical and electroencephalographic study. *J. Neurosurg.* **14**, 249.

Penfield, W. and Jasper, H. (1954). Epilepsy and the functional anatomy of the human brain. Churchill, London.

Penfield, W. and Erickson, T. C. (1941). Epilepsy and cerebral localisation. Thomas, Springfield, Ill.

Penfield, W. and Shaver, M. (1945). *Res. Pub. Ass. Nerv. Ment. Dis.* **24**, 620.

Phillips, G. (1954). Traumatic epilepsy after closed head injury. *J. Neurol Neurosurg. Psychiat.* **17**, 1.

Pott, P. (1759). Observations on nature and consequences of wounds and contusions of the head. London.

Rapport, R. L. and Penry, J. K. (1972). Pharmacologic prophylaxis of post-traumatic epilepsy. *Epilepsia* **13**, 295.

Rapport, R. L. and Penry, J. K. (1973). A survey of attitudes toward the pharmacological prophylaxis of post-traumatic epilepsy. *J. Neurosurg.* **38**, 159.

Reichmann, V. (1927). Ueber Entstehung und Haufigkeit epileptischer Krampfe nach Schadelburchen an der Hand von 603 Fallen. *Deutsche Zischr. f. Nervenh.* **96**, 260.

Renfrew, S., Haggar, I. and Watson, M. (1957). Predictability of the EEG in people with seizures. *Arch. Neurol. Psychiat. (Chicago)* **78**, 329.

Riddoch, G. (1932). Discussion on the diagnosis and treatment of acute head injuries. *Proc. Roy. Soc. Med.* **25**, 735.

Rish, B. L. and Caveness, W. F. (1973). Prophylaxis and the occurrence of early fits in craniocerebral trauma in Vietnam. *J. Neurosurg.* **38**, 155.

Rodin, E. A. (1968). The prognosis of patients with epilepsy. Charles Thomas, Illinois.

Rowbotham, G. F. (1949). Long-term results of injuries of head. *J. ment. Sci.* **95**, 336.

Russell, W. R. (1932). Discussion on the diagnosis and treatment of acute head injuries. *Proc. Roy. Soc. Med.* **25**, 751.

Russell, W. R. (1947). Anatomy of traumatic epilepsy. *Brain* **70**, 225.

Russell, W. R. and Smith, A. (1961). Post-traumatic amnesia in closed head injury. *Arch. Neurol.* **5**, 4.

Russell, W. R. and Whitty, C. W. M. (1952). Studies in traumatic epilepsy. Part I: Facts influencing the incidence of epilepsy after brain wounds. *J. Neurol. Neurosurg. Psychiat.* **15**, 93.

Russell, W. R. and Davies-Jones, G. A. B. (1969). "Epilepsy following the brain wounds of World War II". In: Walker, A. E., Caveness, W. F., Critchley, M. (eds.). The late effects of head injury, Thomas, Springfield.

Sheehan, S. (1958). 1000 cases of late onset epilepsy. *Irish J. Med. Sci.* **390**, 261.

Schou, H. I. (1933). Trauma capitis and epilepsy. *Acta psych. et neurol.* **8**, 75.

Small, J. M. and Woolff, A. L. (1957). Fatal damage to the brain by epileptic convulsions after a trivial injury to the head. *J. Neurol. Neurosurg. Psychiat.* **20**, 293.

Smith, B., Robinson, G. C. and Lennox, W. G. (1954). Acquired epilepsy; study of 535 cases. *Neurology* **4**, 19.

Stöwsand D. (1971). Paresen und epileptische Reaktionen im initialstadium des hirntraumas. G. T. Verlag, Stuttgart.

Stöwsand, D. and Bues, E. (1970). Fruhanfalle unde ihre verlaufe nach hirntraumen im Kindesalter. *Z. Neurol.* **198**, 201.

Stöwsand, D. and Geile, G. (1966). Cerebrale symptome bei impressions frakturen der schadelkonvexität. *Dtsch. Z. Nervenheilk* **186**, 330.

Symonds, C. P. (1935). Traumatic epilepsy. *Lancet* ii, 1217.

Symonds, C. P. (1942). Discussion of differential diagnosis and treatment of post-contusional states. *Proc. Roy. Soc. Med.* **35**, 601.

Symonds, C. (1962). Concussion and its sequelae. *Lancet* i, 1.

Symonds, C. P. and Russell, W. R. (1943). Accidental head injuries. *Lancet* i, 7.

Teather, D. (1974). Diagnosis — methods and analysis. *Bull. Inst. Math. App.* **10**, 37.

Temkin, O. (1945). "The Falling Sickness". John Hopkins Press, Baltimore, U.S.A.

Terespolsky, P. S. (1972). Post-traumatic epilepsy. *Forensic Science* **1**, 147.

Trotter, W. (1924). Certain minor injuries of the brain. *Lancet* i, 935.

Turner, J. W. A. and Eden, K. (1941). Loss of consciousness in different types of head injury. *Proc. Roy. Soc. Med.* **34**, 685.

Vitale, A., Domdey, M. and Remond, A. (1953). Etude EEG de l'epilepsie temporale d'origine traumatique. *Rev. Neurol.* **88**, 374.

Wagstaff, W. W. (1928). The incidence of traumatic epilepsy after gunshot wound of the head. *Lancet* ii, 861.

Walker, A. E. (1956). Natural history of post-traumatic epilepsy. *Trans. Amer. Neurol. Ass.* **81**, 37.

Walker, A. E. (1957). Prognosis in post-traumatic epilepsy. A ten year follow-up of craniocerebral injuries of World War II. *J. Amer. Med. Ass.* **164**, 1636.

Walker, A. E. (1958). In Gurdijan, E. S. and Webster, J. E. (q.v.).

Walker, A. E. and Erculei, F. (1963). The late results of cranioplasty. *Arch. Neurol.* **9**, 105.

Walker, A. E. and Erculei, F. (1968). Head injured men 15 years later. Thomas, Illinois.

Walton, J. N. (1963). Some observations on the value of EEG in medico-legal practice. *Medicolegal Journal* **31**, 15.

Weiss, G. H. and Caveness, W. F. (1972). Prognostic factors in the persistence of post-traumatic epilepsy. *J. Neurosurg.* Vol. **37**, 164.

White, J. C., Liu, C. T. and Mixter, W. J. (1948). Focal epilepsy. II. Epilepsy secondary to cerebral trauma and infection. *New Engl. J. Med.* **239**, 1.

Whitty, C. W. M. (1947). Early traumatic epilepsy. *Brain* **70**, 416.

Williams, D. (1941a). The EEG in acute head injuries. *J. Neurol. Neurosurg. Psychiat.* **4**, 107.

Williams, D. (1941b). The EEG in chronic post-traumatic states. *J. Neurol. Neurosurg. Psychiat.* **4**, 131.

Williams, D. (1944). The electroencephalogram in traumatic epilepsy. *J. Neurol. Neurosurg. Psychiat.* **7**, 103.

Williams, D. (1950). New Orientations in epilepsy. *Brit. Med. J.* i, 685.

Worster-Drought, C. (1961). Medical evidence in personal injury cases by Dix, D. K. and Todd, A. H. Lewis, London.

Wilson, A. K. (1955). Neurology, Butterworth, London.

INDEX